DATE DUE

OCT 1 4 2010		
FEB 1 5 2019		

LIVING WITH LOW VISION AND BLINDNESS

ABOUT THE AUTHORS

John M. Crandell, Jr., Ph.D.

Dr. Crandell became blind at age eight. He attended public school without support services for four years and then transferred to the Arizona State School for the Deaf and the Blind. He attended two years of college before serving two years as the first blind missionary for his church. He returned to and graduated from Arizona State University with a B.A. in education and began teaching in a one room school. He changed careers to rehabilitation teaching and counseling. Later, after obtaining a Master's degree from Arizona State University and a Ph.D. from the University of Texas at Austin in counseling psychology and special education, Dr. Crandell obtained teaching positions at Temple University and Brigham Young University. His tenure at BYU included being Director of Teacher Preparation for Teachers of the Visually Impaired. He served on many national, state, and local advisory committees. He retired from BYU after 25 years as professor of educational psychology and special education.

Lee W. Robinson, Ed.D.

Dr. Robinson began his career in public education. After receiving an M.A. degree from Brigham Young University, he taught in a residential school for the blind, later becoming an administrator and director of federal grants for demonstration projects in early childhood education. Interests in learning theory and his own legal blindness led to further study and graduation with an Ed.D. degree in educational psychology and special education from Brigham Young University. Dr. Robinson is the author of curricula for preschool children, has written many articles, and made many presentations in the field of work for the blind. He was the first president and executive director of the National Association of Parents of the Visually Impaired (NAPVI). He has served on numerous national advisory committees, as an officer in organizations of the blind, and received national recognition awards.

LIVING WITH LOW VISION AND BLINDNESS

Guidelines That Help Professionals and Individuals Understand Vision Impairments

By

JOHN M. CRANDELL, Jr., Ph.D.

and

LEE W. ROBINSON, Ed.D.

CHARLES C THOMAS • PUBLISHER, LTD.
Springfield • Illinois • U.S.A.

Published and Distributed Throughout the World by

CHARLES C THOMAS • PUBLISHER, LTD.
2600 South First Street
Springfield, Illinois 62704

©2007 by CHARLES C THOMAS • PUBLISHER, LTD.

ISBN 978-0-398-07741-9 (hard)
ISBN 978-0-398-07742-6 (paper)

Library of Congress Catalog Card Number: 2007003435

With THOMAS BOOKS *careful attention is given to all details of man-*
ufacturing and design. It is the Publisher's desire to present books that are sat-
isfactory as to their physical qualities and artistic possibilities and appropri-
ate for their particular use. THOMAS BOOKS *will be true to those laws*
of quality that assure a good name and good will.

Printed in the United States of America
CR-R-3

Library of Congress Cataloging-in-Publication Data

Crandell, John M.
  Living with low vision and blindness : guidelines that help professionals and individuals
understand vision impairments / by John M. Crandell, Jr. and Lee W. Robinson.
    p. ; cm.
  Includes bibliographical references and index.
  ISBN-13: 978-0-398-07741-9 (hard cover)
  ISBN-10: 0-398-07741-X (hard cover)
  ISBN-13: 978-0-398-07742-6 (pbk.)
  ISBN-10: 0-398-07742-8 (pbk.)
  1. Vision disorders. 2. People with visual disabilities--Rehabilitation. 3. Blindness--
Patients--Rehabilitation. I. Robinson, Lee W. II. Title.
  [DNLM: 1. Blindness--psychology. 2. Blindness--rehabilitation. 3. Vision, Low--psycholo-
gy. 4. Vision, Low--rehabilitation. 5. Visually Impaired Persons--psychology. 6. Visually
Impaired Persons--rehabilitation. WW 276 C891L 2007]
  RE91.C73 2007
  617.7--dc22
                                                              2007003435

PREFACE

Will Rogers is credited with the statement "Everyone talks about the weather but nobody does anything about it." We feel that, like the weather, there is a lot of discussion about education and rehabilitation services to the blind, but often there are feelings of discouragement about efforts to overcome poor quality services or the lack of services. This book is an effort to review some past discussions, suggest ways to improve and increase the amount of services available to those who are blind or who have low vision.

Hopefully, those who have been trained as educators or rehabilitation specialists in the field of work for the blind and visually impaired will find information that is new or that will remind them of issues which still need to be resolved. However, **this book is meant to be an overview of issues which need to be understood by psychologists, social workers, educators, rehabilitation specialists, therapists, families, and others who have little or no training in work for the blind and visually impaired.** Others will find information from the fields of general psychology, science, and regular education we have encountered which could prove helpful in understanding and improving services to those who are blind or who have low vision.

We have departed somewhat from traditional scholarship in that specific references are not cited. What is discussed here comes from texts, journal articles, and many years of experience in work for the blind and visually impaired. References consist of only a few books and articles listed after each chapter as "Suggested Readings." Many of these will lead readers to in-depth study of subjects of interest to them. Other sources which are listed provide a rich background for understanding the needs and complexities of providing education and rehabilitation services to this very diverse, low incident population. The population consists of children, students and adults who never have had or who have lost most or all of their eyesight. Some readings are not still used in professional training programs because of the limited time available to professors to present vast amounts of information needed to serve the array of children, students and clients. We consider most of the suggested readings to be vintage material that should be considered by those interested in serving the blind and visually impaired.

Our viewpoint is that absence of or the loss of the sense of sight makes individuals who are "blind" different to the degree that quality services are most likely to be provided by professionals and agencies that have special training and experience. This perspective seems at odds with the current general philosophy and current practices, services, and programs. For several decades, state and federal funding patterns, professional training, and public misunderstanding of the effects of vision loss have pushed services toward a "one size fits all" approach. We believe when concept development, self-concept, motivation, perception, emotions and attitudes are impacted by loss or absence of sight to the degree they are, that specialized programs and services are the most effective and efficient way to help the individual be a productive, independent and contented member of their community. We also believe that contributions from science, medicine, psychology, and sociology provide information about neurology, memory, psychological adjustment, and engineering that can be used to serve the blind and visually impaired better.

The ways individuals who are blind or have low vision accommodate, learn and perform successfully are not in any way inferior to other ways, just different. Neither are the methods of instruction, things to be learned and adaptive technology inferior, just different. Hopefully the material presented here will help bring understanding to the differences and suggest improvements professionals trained to work with the blind and visually impaired as well as those from other professions can make.

It is not expected that all will agree with what is presented here. It is hoped that due consideration will be given to the views and information. It is hoped that this book will benefit individuals wishing to provide programs and services for those who are blind or who have low vision.

John M. Crandell, Jr.
Lee W. Robinson

INTRODUCTION

The educational and rehabilitation systems for blind and partially seeing persons (along with all special education and rehabilitation services) are in a state of great flux. There is no consensus of where the upheaval will lead, whether toward greater inclusion of these persons into the educational and vocational "mainstream" or toward more isolated programs, or toward something quite different.

There is a need to consider the progress the fields of blind education and rehabilitation have made in the centuries since Valentin Hauy began the process of preparing those without sight for participation in the broader society. There have been controversies throughout the years and, hopefully, we have learned something from the resolution of these difficulties. Several excellent books have offered some viewpoints on these difficulties (e.g. Koestler, 1986; Scholl, 1986).

This book is an attempt to summarize the findings in the fields of general education and psychology as they relate to vision loss. It makes no claims of being complete. Hopefully, it will stimulate thought and discussion on some of the issues which face us in this time of great change.

A properly made convex lens increases the apparent size and detail of an object being viewed. The greater the power of a convex lens, the larger the object appears and more of the detail is visible—as with telescopes and microscopes. There is a price which is paid for the increase of size and detail: the field of vision is decreased and the relationship of the detail to the whole is diminished or lost.

In like manner, when emphasis is placed on specific remedial and instructional techniques without the broader perspective provided by theory and principles, the professional worker may not be able to see how a specific program impacts the total life of individuals with vision loss. In the same way, if one becomes so caught up in philosophical and theoretical perspectives, practical concerns of how tasks can be performed may be lost.

A balance between general perspectives and specific intervention approaches needs to be maintained if the lives of those with whom one works are to be properly assisted. It is not enough that an individual client or student knows braille, typing, and travel skills; he/she must also know about the broader society into which he/she needs to enter and to become an independent and contributing member.

This book is designed to provide both a Gestalt or overall perspective in the field of work with the blind and visually impaired and to focus the attention of the reader on the many detailed facets examined in other sources. Vision loss does not occur in isolation from personal and environmental factors, and on the basis of theories, a worker can infer special needs. If these psychological and sociological perspectives are lost, the professional worker will find it difficult to guide the educational and rehabilitative processes for an individual. For example, one area of need for people, including those with vision loss, is to be able to access the environment. Helping a particular visually limited person in meeting this need is not a simple matter of choosing from among several options—sighted guide, guide dog, the long cane, etc. Rather, the professional needs to know about the person's history of vision loss such as age at onset; residual vision, if any; type of loss—central loss or peripheral loss—type of residential area including where the visually impaired person needs to go; family attitudes toward independent travel for their visually limited family member, physical capabilities of the person, including additional disabilities, and so forth before a choice is made. Without the broader perspective, however, there is a strong tendency to focus too narrowly on strictly technical aspects of the program. With a broader perspective, details of the plan for a specific person can be woven into the total pattern.

The book is concerned primarily with providing understanding of the many elements which must be considered before a successful rehabilitative and/or an educational program can be developed. This type of understanding will be illustrated in the pages of the book by examples drawn from experience which the authors have observed directly. Theoretical factors will be described which must be considered in the development of a suitable program for a person with specific strengths and weaknesses.

Discussions will also be included related to the meaning and implications of self-concept and self-esteem in the overall adjustment of individuals with vision loss. We will also evaluate psychological and sociological theories of "the blind" as described in writings such as Kim's, *The Community of the Blind*, and Scott's, *The Making of Blind Men*, in terms of their relevance to life adjustment. An attempt will be made to identify weaknesses in the research bases in this field and propose specific research activities which could help alleviate problems.

Another focus will be provision of explanations of the origin, development, influence, and modification of public attitudes toward blindness and the influence of these attitudes on the adjustment of individuals with blindness. We will use information—concepts and theories—in the development of specific goals and objectives for a specific person with unique characteristics in a service setting: writing an "IWRP" or "IEP."

This book is foundational, i.e., providing a framework within which to fit materials from many sources. The knowledge base for this book consists of the historical and research literature available in texts, and from the professional journals. An attempt has been made to organize this book on the basis of a systematic and reasoned outline to provide scaffolding upon which the content of theories can be place. It starts with simple ideas and moves toward more complex concepts. Suggested Readings are given after each chapter as well as at the end of this preface.

SUGGESTED READINGS

1. Koestler, Francis A. (1976). The unseen minority: A social history of blindness in the United States. New York: David McKay Company, Inc.
2. Scholl, G.T. (1986). *Foundations of education for blind and visually handicapped children and youth: Theory and practice.* New York: American Foundation for the Blind.
3. Scott, R.A. (1968). *The making of blind men.* New York: Russell Sage Foundation.

ACKNOWLEDGMENTS

Any contribution the authors may make to help individuals who are blind or who have low vision as well as professionals in the field of work with this population is heavily indebted to many generations of leaders and dedicated teachers and rehabilitation workers who have devoted their lives to service for the blind and visually impaired. We have had the opportunity to become personally acquainted with many of these individuals and have benefitted from their efforts. Likewise, there are many current friends and colleagues who have encouraged and supported us during our many years of work. We express our deep appreciation to each and all of them.

Our families have also supported and labored along with us to see that this book has been completed. Without their support and tolerance, it would not have been possible to spend long hours of discussion and writing. We hope they will be pleased and rewarded for their consistent encouragement.

CONTENTS

LIVING WITH LOW VISION
AND BLINDNESS

Chapter 1

CURRENT SETTING

There are many speculative opinions about how individuals who are blind or who have low vision may be different from those who have normal or correctable eyesight. There are just as many opinions about how individuals with visually impairments are the same as other people. Perhaps the more important question is, "What evidence is there to support either side of the arguments?" Amidst all the questions and opinions, "What difference does it make to the person with blindness or low vision?"

Founders of programs of education and rehabilitation for the blind and visually impaired have been divided over these issues since the first schools for the blind were begun in the late eighteenth and early nineteenth centuries. Early examples of successful blind individuals seemed to point to unusual abilities which should be fostered through specialized education, training, and support. Other notable pioneers stressed that the blind should be included in the "common" schools and receive the same curricula as their sighted peers. The different philosophies have spawned controversy for over two centuries and continues today with most avid debaters shedding more heat than light on the issues.

General changes in society have had their influences on the prevalence of segregated or integrated programs for the blind. For example, during most of the 1800s only a few programs were supported outside of special schools for the blind. This reflected the general attitude of society toward all those who were disabled. Asylums, poor houses, and orphanages were the major alternatives to total support from the family, usually in an agrarian setting. Thoughts of alternative ways to provide for the blind/visually impaired shifted to more local community-based efforts as the populist movement began to advocate for services that would meet the needs of a more industrialized society. This general change split the field of work for the blind. There were those who strongly advocated for the continuation of state-supported schools and eleemosynary institutions. There were equally strong advocates who stressed the importance of being in the "world of the seeing." Each pointed with pride to the successes of those completing their programs.

One common theme through the decades of debate has been the assumption and belief that, given the appropriate education or vocational training, individuals who are blind or have low vision can be successful and happy adults who participate in and contribute to society. The success, however, has often depended upon the willingness of society to provide resources including specially trained personnel, adaptive equipment, and equal opportunities for gainful employment. Governmental funding has waxed and waned with the nation's economy and the corollary meant that the disabled were the last to be hired and the first to be fired.

As an example, during the era of post World War II, the costs of war and the influx of women into the work force as well as the return of military personnel to civilian pursuits made it difficult for those who were blind to obtain employment even when well educated and qualified. This situation was observed by governmental entities and rehabilitation programs were begun that emphasized employment in "new" occupations. Orientation and mobility programs, which were first begun to aid returning veterans, became a part of training in virtually all rehabilitation agencies. By the 1960s, the United States was in an economic position to support many more special programs as a part of the " Great Society." Many professional personnel training program were in operation. Later, as the national economy worsened, many programs lost funding and closed or were severely limited in scope.

Beginning with the Rehabilitation Act of 1973, and the Education for All Handicapped Children Act of 1975, and extending until the present, another cycle has been evident. These two public laws of the United States have entitled those with disabilities, including those who are blind/visually impaired, to education and rehabilitation with the expectation that given opportunities they would be integrated into society. In early stages of implementation, many new programs were begun and both state and federal efforts provided considerable new funding. However, again as the economic tides shifted, Congress did not fund programs as "promised" and many unfunded mandates have stretched the resources to a point where the quality and effectiveness of services being provided has come into question with a corresponding skepticism about the value of special education in general with concerns that spill-over into services for the blind. The need for unique services to the blind is especially under fire.

The laws which have generated current special education and rehabilitation programs are mostly based on an "inclusion" philosophy giving extreme preference to participation in the "general" programs. Funding patterns at the national and state level have supported this philosophy to almost the total exclusion of all other models of service. Providers of specialized services are being forced to provide evidence that there is a need for specialized services to the blind and those with severe low vision. The predominant models support generic programs even though the facts provide evidence that two-thirds of the workforce of eligible blind are unemployed or underemployed, which would indicate lack of success of the generic approach. So, the speculation and debate about whether special or generic models of service best meet the needs of individuals who are blind or who have low vision continues.

Blind Persons Are Different

One factor that continues to fire debates as to whether the blind are more like than different from the sighted is the diversity of the population. As will be discussed in later chapters, the blind are found among all social and economic strata of society. It does not matter whether families are rich or poor, whether they come from a specific geographic region, whether they descend from any particular racial or ethnic background; all are touched by loss of sight. This may be from having an infant born into the family who is blind or it may be the result of disease or accident any time later in life. Fortunately, the number of those who are blind or have severe low vision is relatively small, but this, too, makes identifying and understanding the needs through valid and reliable research difficult.

Until the inventions of modern imaging techniques that allow observations of brain activity in humans, researchers could only speculate about what happens when the sense of sight is not ever present or when it is lost. From animal studies, researchers found that the brains of rats changed when eyes were removed with the visual centers becoming smaller and other areas increasing in size. Monkeys and cats placed in environments that had only one visual pattern available to them were later unable to detect other patterns. While these were interesting findings, it was not possible to confirm similar findings in humans. However, folk lore, such as blind people have a better sense of hearing or touch, seemed to make sense. These studies suggested to some how the brain of blind individuals might function in different ways from the sighted. Conclusions from these animal studies stressed the unique features blindness has on neural development.

Studies by professionals using techniques that measured the sensitivity of hearing and touch seemed to refute any notions that brain functions of the blind were different. Measured acuities of the senses did not support ideas that the blind were different except they could not see. Likewise, those with other disabilities have more characteristics like "normal" children than not. This "evidence" was used by advocates of generic philosophies to support *their* service models designed to "mainstream" students or clients.

Still, regardless of how grounded service providers are in generic services for the blind even those grounded in the generic models must recognize that some tasks such as concept formation are supported by visual stimuli. In fact, some concepts such as color, clouds, flames, and other phenomena are not possible for those with total absence of sight to understand in the same fashion as individuals with sight do. So, questions about the differences between individuals who are blind and those with sight persist. How do those who are blind form concepts? Are the same centers in the brain used to store and retrieve information? Are tactile stimuli as powerful or can they replace visual input effectively? The fact that adaptations to the learning media are needed for training make it obvious that different centers of the brain will be involved. Tactile media surely require that tactile areas of the brain be more active. Taking advantage of the brain's plasticity to learn would seem to require those who provide services to study special theories and methods unique to the blind.

In the past few years, magnetic resonance imaging which allow observation of electrical activity in the brain without surgical invasion has shown that "image centers" in the brain are different when children are born without sight and change when sight is lost later in life. It seems that the plasticity of the brain allows centers which normally would accept and respond to visual stimuli to change and serve other functions. This seems to confirm that changes similar to those found in animal studies occur in humans when the need for adaptation is present and humans seem to have much more ability to change. The evidence is clear that sight loss causes changes in brain functions. What is known should be used to develop instructional methods best suited to different neurological capacities.

Blindness Makes All the Difference

As indicated in the opening of this chapter, professionals in the field of work for the blind have been deeply divided over how different the blind are from the sighted. Those who felt there were significant differences engaged in trying to demonstrate the difference through discussion of a "psychology of blindness." The latest neurological information shows evidence of significant differences between sighted and blind individuals. This supports the need for a psychology of blindness.

Many of the writings of earlier eras that discussed psychological development of the blind, which were once studied as a part of professional training, have been taken from the curriculum. Most of today's teachers, counselors, orientation and mobility instructors, psychologist, and other support personnel have not taken an opportunity to consider whether a separate "psychology" is helpful to work for the blind. This book is an effort to have anyone interested in blindness and low vision consider how individuals who are blind receive sensory input, use memory and association processes to form concepts, and how their lives are influenced by different organic as well as social differences.

Each experience of a blind person is unique to that individual. No one single theory or set of experiences has proven to account for all success or all failure of individuals who are blind. It should be understood that even with the instrumentation that seems to allow scientists to "observe" what is happening inside the skull, such factors as how associations are made, what motivates individuals, how choices are made, and many other functions of the mind are not understood. Only electrical activity is being observed, but the causes and relationships are not shown. The factors such as motivation and volition, though not well understood, definitely are a part of the psychology for all individuals. How they may or may not be influenced by lack of sight is not understood any better in those who are blind than for those with normal eyesight. It will be evident to readers that the authors of this work believe that blindness creates unique needs for specialized services and that those who provide such services need a deep understanding of the physiological and psychological differences between those who have normal eyesight and those who do not.

The purpose of this book is *not* to be neutral on the issues discussed but rather to use information from general psychology and other fields to illustrate how the theories and services effect the lives of blind people. It is expected that not everyone will agree with the suggested conclusions reached by the authors. It is hoped that what is discussed will cause thoughtful consideration of the impact of blindness, especially in the education and rehabilitation processes.

The uniqueness of being blind is in no way inferior to "normal," simply different. Those who are blind as well as those with any other disability must not be regarded as second-class citizens. Through appropriate training and education, as well as learning through interaction with the physical and social environments, individuals who are blind can and do become self-sufficient, caring, and contributing members of society.

Chapter 2

CONCEPT DEVELOPMENT

In this chapter, there will be a foundation laid for the rest of the text in the form of a cognitive framework. This framework identifies some of the assumptions underlying the approach to special education in general and the education and programs for persons with visually impairments/handicaps in particular.

Although the concepts described here are philosophical in nature, and the terminology is probably unfamiliar, the ideas are *not* difficult and have relevance for many other aspects of life. If readers will take the time and expend the energy necessary to become thoroughly conversant with these ideas (even if they do not agree with them), it will clarify other concepts presented later.

The world in which people live is extremely complex and there is little agreement about its nature. Cognitive theory offers an approach to the study of the world and all that is in it. This theory holds that people deal with the diversity and details of the world by organizing experiences into categories or concepts. In these categories, objects, persons and events are grouped into collected entities so they can more easily be dealt with by using concepts. It is easier to interact with these groupings instead of dealing with all of the objects, persons, and events as though each one is unique (which, in fact, they are). Trees, for example, are each different in some respects from one another, but they can be put into the category of trees, and to a limited extent, all of them can be dealt with in similar or completely common ways.

OBJECTIVES

At the completion of this chapter the reader should be able to:

1. Define the terms concept and attribute and demonstrate understanding of the relationship between them.
2. Distinguish between concepts based upon criterial, functional, and formal attributes.
3. Describe the hierarchal structure of concepts into superordinate, coordinate, and subordinate levels and how these allow people to organize their world for easier storage and retrieval of information about it.

THE NATURE OF CONCEPTS

The story is told of the farmer who hired a worker to help around the farm while the farmer, himself, took care of other business matters. The first day, the farmer assigned the worker to clean out the barn. At the end of the day, when the farmer returned home, he was pleased to find that the barn was thoroughly cleaned and organized.

The second day, the worker was sent to plow a specific field. Like the barn cleaning, the farmer expected this task would take several days. But when he returned, he found the job done very well.

The next two days, other assignments were completed with the same efficiency as the first two. The farmer, thinking that he had asked too much of his hired hand, decided to give him an easier task on the fifth day so he told him to sort a big pile of potatoes into three piles: a pile of large, a pile of medium, and a pile of small potatoes. When he returned at the end of the day, he found only a small portion of the pile divided up.

"I don't understand," he said to the hired hand. "You had done so well on the other tasks, I thought you would find this task a break for you." "The job was not hard," answered the hired hand. "What took so long was making the decisions."

One of the major problems faced in life is properly organizing and classifying objects, persons, and events which are encountered. The broad categories are not hard to understand, but when the learner gets down to specifics, then there are difficulties in assigning experiences to their rightful categories. This usually stems from the use of poorly defined concepts where the defining attributes are not clearly observable.

In a rough way, languages are heavily involved in this problem. Almost all nouns and pronouns represent labels assigned to the various categories or groupings in the world. Adjectives help define differences in groupings which are similar. For example, one will ask for the "blue" book to help separate it from the category of "red" books. Sometimes these adjectives are themselves not sufficient so they need further subdivisions such as "dark blue" books, or "bright red" books.

As of several years ago, biologists had identified over five million living species of animals. This included all of the subspecies as well as the broad categories of reptiles, mammals, insects, fish, etc. Some species which were identifiable on the basis of characteristics which are clearly observed by the senses, were further divided into subspecies on the basis of unobservable, underlying characteristics such as common genetic materials–DNA, for example.

Those species classified on the basis of surface or easily observed qualities are referred to as "phenotypes." Those species identified and classified on the basis of unobservable qualities are called "genotypes."

To illustrate, dinosaurs are assumed to have been part of the class of animals called reptiles. One property of reptiles is that they have no body "thermostat" so their blood temperatures would vary as outside temperatures changed instead of the relatively constant 98.6 degrees fahrenheit humans have for that temperature. Birds are assumed to have evolved from reptiles, including dinosaurs, but birds are "warm blooded." This has led some scientists to question whether birds came from reptiles or whether some reptiles, including dinosaurs, may have been warm blooded, too. In any event, scientists cannot go out and observe directly whether dinosaurs have warm or cold blood since no dinosaurs are around to observe and their bones do not provide evidence one way or the other. Presumably, birds possess certain underlying structural features which some scientists see as evidence for this classification.

In much the same way, observers classify persons on the basis of age, size, brightness, temperament, etc. They distinguish children from adults on the basis of age and size, but what about other qualities? Do children differ from adults on the basis of brightness, or temperament, etc.? Some children are larger than some adults. Some children even seem to look older than some adults. If the age of a person is not known, it is sometimes difficult to make a proper classification. In other words, the boundary between the concepts "children" and "adult" are ambiguous. It is at these boundaries that difficulties with categories arise. For the huge majority of cases, a person does not have difficulty in categorizing children and adults easily.

CONCEPT DEVELOPMENT

The world in which people live is so complex that human beings, cannot cope with it if every experience were to be treated as though it were unique (which, in fact, it is). It is, therefore, necessary to observe similarities and differences among objects, events, and persons and to group these elements together into categories. This does not imply that all exemplars or elements in a category are identical. Nor does it mean that an element can be categorized into only one class or group. People are all a part of many groups or communities, e.g., male or female; old, middle-aged, or young; American, English, Mexican; Republicans, Democrats, Independents; Catholic, Protestant, Mormon, Jew; members of a profession; residents of a state or community.

To identify (or classify) a person as being visually impaired should carry no supposition that all other classes are excluded as additional groupings into which a person can be placed. There can be a strong presupposition, however, that there are some other groups which are appropriate, i.e., groups of persons who will have difficulty in mobility, getting access to printed materials, developing some concepts, etc. There is even a better-than-chance probability that a person classified as visually impaired will also be a member of such groups as the poor, the unemployed, and hard-of-hearing.

Although loss of sight is not a desirable condition, and although it places many burdens on the person experiencing vision loss, it is a condition which, with appropriate help, can be lived with in a rewarding and productive fashion. This text, along with other writings and experiences, will help prepare the reader to give that special help.

ATTRIBUTES

An attribute is a quality, characteristic, trait, property, or feature possessed or attributed to an object, person, or event. There are several types of attributes: criterial, functional, and formal, for example. It is the set of these attributes which describes or distinguishes the group's concepts, classes, or categories used in understanding the world and the many elements in it.

Criterial attributes are those which can be directly observed by our senses, viz., colors, shapes, sizes, locations, movements. Objects are described in terms of their colors, i.e., black shoes, blue skies, gray fog, tall men. Concepts based on criterial attributes are the first groupings used by children. These categories are very useful and easily developed. There are other kinds of attributes which characterize more complex aspects of the world. One kind is functional attributes.

Functional attributes are terms which allow for the grouping together in the same category of objects which are obviously different in terms of criterial attributes. For example, the observer groups together pens, pencils, chalk, typewriters, computers, quills, braille slates as "writing instruments." Pens, pencils, chalk, and quills share some criterial attributes, but typewriters, computers, and braille slates are very different from other writing equipment. It is the common use or function of all these and other writing instruments which makes it possible to see them as sharing their position in this grouping.

Still more complex aspects of the world are grouped together on the basis of relationships. For example, the concept "uncle" is different from those of "writing instrument" or "red books." Uncles are males who have a brother or sister who in turn has a child. They may have many brothers and/or sisters who have many children. But it is the relationships involved which establishes the classification of uncle.

Other abstract categories are also based on the use of "formal attributes." The term "formal" comes from the field of logic and refers to relationships. Three other kinds of attributes are important. These are "defining attributes," "noisy attributes," and "quiet attributes." The sets of attributes which describe or characterize the objects, persons, or events to be placed in a particular category are referred to as defining attributes. If properly developed, the set of such attributes should unambiguously distinguish one concept from all other concepts. It is possible to use only one attribute for a specific concept, but such a concept would include only a very small number of exemplars, or it would include far too many exemplars with greatly diminished utility. As noted above, the use of the attribute "black" to define a large group of persons ignores too many other attributes which can usefully distinguish among those with dark skin. When it is assumed that all those with black skin also share many or all other attributes, one commits the error of stereotype. Although a stereotype is economical in that it does not require careful observations, it can result in improperly assuming that all those with the stereotypical attribute are all of a kind.

An attribute which is used to form a stereotype is referred to as a "noisy" attribute. This one or a small number of attributes can limit the effectiveness of the effort to understand the world. The color of an automobile may be a strongly attractive property of an automobile, but it is almost worthless in judging the quality of an efficient transportation entity. Noisy attributes call attention to an object, person, or event but lack utility in making it possible for one to understand the world.

"Quiet" attributes are similarly restricted in usefulness because they are shared by many other concepts, categories, or groups. Thus, the statement that disabled children are more like normal children than they are different is true, but they are more alike because they share attributes which do not allow for specific educational planning and methods. Children who are intellectually impaired breathe, walk, eat, and smile as do children of normal intelligence, but this observation alone does not help in preparing an educational program for children with low I.Q. or limited intellectual ability.

There are other kinds of attributes and concepts, but these few clarifications provide examples which will guide in the analysis of concepts. The reader will be able to see how the use of improper categorizing attributes confuses language and allows the creation of stereotypes and "scapegoats" which complicate social relations. The use of the attribute "black" and the assumption that ALL black persons possess all attributes in common has led to great injustices. In like manner, the assumption that all persons classified as "blind" are all alike or the assumption that ALL persons who have a disability are alike, overly simplifies the highly complex problems of assisting such persons in contributing to the world's progress.

DEFINITION OF BLINDNESS

If readers were to look up the definition of "blindness" in a dictionary or encyclopedia, they will note particular generalizations made about those with vision loss. In order to establish eligibility for services, educational, rehabilitative, or financial assistance, it has been necessary to establish a "legal definition" of blindness. This definition is: Visual acuity of 20/200 or less in the better eye with best correction; or, visual acuity of better than 20/200, but with a restricted field of vision which subtends an angle of 20 degrees.

(Someone has suggested that a definition of "illegal" blindness is exemplified by politicians. It is claimed that they are lacking in insight, foresight, vision and perspective; they do not learn from hindsight; they suffer from oversight, shortsightedness microscopy, and lack of farsightedness. They have a muddled outlook, and their perceptual windows are closed.)

This definition is based on the ability of the normal eye to see letters or figures of standard sizes at a specified distance, usually 20 feet or the equivalent. The term "acuity" is used to describe the "sharpness" of vision in terms of a fraction like expression, the numerator refers to the distance at which the individual subject is tested, and the denominator-like part of the expression refers to the distance at which a normal or average eye can see a particular letter, number, or figure.

A second part of the definition indicates that a person may have better vision than is allowed by the first part of the definition if there is a defect in the visual field or breadth of vision which is less than 20 degrees.

As an example of this definition with which most people are familiar, normal vision is described as 20/20. This means that the average person, at a distance of 20 feet, is able to read the size of figure which that average person can see at 20 feet. If, on the other hand, a person is tested at 20 feet and can see no better than the letter which is seen by the normal or average person at 40 feet, then his/her vision would be described as 20/40 visual acuity.

The upper limit of legal blindness is the ability to see at 20 feet the figure which the normal person can see at 200 feet. A person with visual acuity between 20/70 and 20/200 is usually classified as partially sighted, and in most cases, will need specialized assistance, though such a person would probably be able to read newsprint at a reduced distance.

Within the definition of blindness, there are many subdivisions or groups. Between 10 percent and 20 percent of persons who are legally blind have no useful vision. Another group can see light, but no detail. Still others can see shadows or hand movements against a lighted background.

There are differences in the ability of one who has useful vision with respect to how he/she uses that residual vision. For example, a person with visual acuity of 20/200 may be able to read normal print in a book at a reduced distance or with a magnifier. The type of eye condition which has produced the vision loss will also be involved. For example, a person with no or limited central vision may have good peripheral vision and still have difficulty reading print without special aids. This person would most likely have no difficulty in independent travel, while a person with residual central vision but with restricted field vision could probably read print but would have difficulty in independent travel, especially at night.

There are many attributes which can be used for the development of subcategories of legal blindness such as: age at onset of vision defect; type of condition which has produced the visual defect; training or experience with use of limited vision; central vs. peripheral losses; kinds of things which can be seen under varying light and other conditions; level of sensitivity to light; level of acuity; and so forth. The presence of additional disabilities can also affect the ability to use residual vision. Intellectual ability and academic achievement also influence vision use. Some individuals may have considerable as well as very useful remaining vision, but their eyes may fatigue easily, thus limiting the amount of time and the kinds of tasks for which that vision may be used. If a person has the use of only one eye, this can further impact the ways in which residual vision may be used.

Many "low-vision aids" have been developed to assist persons with limited vision make efficient use of remaining vision. These range from simple hand-held magnifiers to closed circuit television devices which can alter the size and color/contrast of the materials to be viewed. The motivation and need for such aids are important factors. The costs and usefulness of such devices also influence whether the devices are obtained and used.

Registries and databases on the blind do not typically collect and organize information about these many subgroups, though research studies often cite the need for more homogeneous subgroups as they attempt to interpret research data. The database kept by the American Printing House for the Blind has provided evidence of national trends and support for the development of programs and materials. A similar national and expanded database could identify potential research subjects with various characteristics important in research and would be most useful and would increase the ability to meet the educational, vocational, social, and personal quality of life issues for those with vision loss.

IMPAIRMENT, DISABILITY, HANDICAP

Readers will find in the same sources as in the section above, the root meanings of the words "impairment," "disability," and "handicap." It is interesting to speculate about why these terms have been used interchangeably by most persons, including those in special education and/or rehabilitation.

Godfrey Stevens, a Professor of Special Education and Rehabilitation at the University of Pittsburgh, in his doctoral dissertation, discussed and clarified the meanings and uses of the terms "impairment,""disability," and "handicap." A careful reading of his work and adoption of the terms as he defined them would do much to clarify communication between and among professionals in rehabilitation and special education. Historically, the terms have been used interchangeably as philosophies have changed and people wished to be "politically" correct. Readers should be aware of these changes as they study professional literature.

The term "impairment" refers to any diseased, disordered, or missing body organ tissues. Among impairments would be brain tissues which do not perform the function of transmitting nerve impulses to an appropriate region of the brain because the chemical transmitters are not produced or have been altered by a genetic defect, hair missing from the head of a man, a finger cut off by a knife, pancreatic beta cells which do not produce insulin, lung tissues which have been attacked by a virus, and so forth.

The diagnosis and treatment of impairments are essentially medical concerns. Examples of interventions for impairments would be the prescription of lenses for reading, the purchase of a toupé for baldness, or other medications for combating infections.

The term "disability" is the negation of the term "able." Each body organ is designed to perform one or more functions or tasks. If one of these organs is unable to perform one or more of these tasks either because of an impairment or because the task performance has not ben learned, then that organ is disabled. It can be seen that the inability to perform a function may or may not be the result of an impairment. A child may not be able to read because of diseased brain tissues, from improper teaching methods, from low intelligence, or from lack of exposure to reading instruction. The emphasis is upon the inability of the specific body organ to perform normally expected functions rather than physiological conditions.

The term "handicap" is derived from an ancient practice of selecting potential lucky "charms" by placing one's "hand into a cap" where the charms were placed. The term is applied to a special burden of "extra" strokes a golf player carries when playing with less able players or the extra weight a superior racehorse carries in a race with slower horses. In these cases, the "burden" is designed to "level" the "playing field" to make the competition fairer.

According to Stevens, in education, the term refers to special burdens or difficulties an individual carries or faces, usually the result of an impairment and/or disability. There is no implication of "leveling the playing field" for workers or learners with special problems. Rather, specific burdens (handicaps) are identified which interfere with the attainment of educational, vocational, or social goals. Stevens identified specific kinds of handicaps such as communication, social interactions, concept attainment, and motility, which indicate both physical and mental movement. Other subgroups of handicaps could include transition from school to the workplace, daily living skills, and skill obsolescent. By employing the subcategories of handicaps it is possible to focus on specific difficulties the person with a disability may be facing. For example, the handicap of communication could be subdivided into receptive and expressive communications. Receptive handicaps could be subdivided into inability to read, to see written materials, difficulty in hearing spoken language, and so on.

With these more specific kinds of handicaps, the professional can provide a more specific solution to the problem of alleviating the handicap. Thus, the person who is not able to see the printed page could be provided with recorded materials, braille books and magazines, synthetic speech with computer-based text, and sighted readers. An individual who was unable to hear spoken language could have his/her handicap lessened by provision of training in sign language and/or speech reading.

Perhaps in the fields of special education and rehabilitation, so much emphasis has been placed on the identification of impairments and disabilities that there has been a neglect of the processes which can lift the burdens or handicaps which are borne by those the schools and/or agencies attempt to serve.

A TAXONOMY FOR INDIVIDUALS
WITH LEARNING PROBLEMS

A taxonomy is a way of categorizing or classifying events, persons, or actions. Readers might try to develop a "taxonomy" for students who have learning difficulties or problems in school which does not use physical, mental, or sensory attributes. In other words, develop a categorical system which is different than the traditional basis for special education. (Hint: Instead of looking at characteristics of the learner, consider methods which could be used for remediation.)

A taxonomy is a scientific classification system designed to guide observations or study. In both rehabilitation and special education the traditional classification or categorization system has been built upon differences in physical, mental, sensory, or emotional characteristics of the clients or students. In recent times this taxonomy has come under severe criticism. One criticism is that the categories have been too rigid, leading to " hardening of the categories," which denied services to some individuals because they shared characteristics with two different groupings or stereotypes based on a single attribute such as race. Thus, blind persons who were also mentally retarded or blind children who were also deaf were sometimes not provided the kinds and quality of services they needed. In short, it was argued that categories should be "pure" with all members of the category possessing all of the characteristics of others in that grouping. This type of category or concept is called a "conjunctive" concept. In fairness to these critics, this desire for conjunctive categories was all too often real.

As a result of this criticism, a "noncategorical" system was proposed This movement argued that a simple instructional approach based on principles of behavior modification or reinforcement strategies could be used to modify the behaviors of any person, regardless of physical, mental, sensory-deficits, or emotional disturbances. Individuals who were mentally retarded and learning disabled were placed into a single group or system which made only one distinction between them: either they had specific learning disabilities or they possessed generalized learning disabilities.

The common treatment was to establish a "token economy" in which specific ineffective behaviors were changed through application of varying "schedules of reinforcements." Thus, the solution for individual differences was basically a single methodology based on behavioral theory.

Another approach which hoped to avoid the emphasis on "pure categories" was to emphasize the "common attributes" shared by all children, and to largely ignore the "differences." It has been argued that there are general principles of education and/or rehabilitation counseling which, if properly practiced, would produce essentially the same results regardless of a few "minor" differences. In this approach all children are directed to a single outcome. Categories are eliminated because the goal is the same regardless of differences and/or methods used to attain them.

Another aspect of a "generic" approach is a philosophical assumption that by developing common attributes, social conflicts could be reduced, and social harmony increased. It was argued that "we're down on what we're not up on." If black and white, deaf and blind, learning disabled and mentally retarded persons were to get to know one another, they would form a generalized, coherent society in which common characteristics were foundational, and disruptive and divisive attributes would be downplayed. This form of generic education depends on a common setting for education, the neighborhood school as an example. So, three educational approaches have been and are used in attempts to escape the difficulties of addressing the burdens faced by individual students: a single methodology, a single set of goals, and single type of educational setting.

Although these alternative approaches have been widely applied, there is little sound empirical evidence supporting their efficacy. Most research has typically assessed differences and similarities in the opinions held by various groups of professional workers or the relatives of clients/students.

Perhaps a more reasonable solution to the problems associated with the use of conjunctive categories would be to use "disjunctive" groupings. Disjunctive concepts are those in which exemplars of a given category share one or more of the defining attributes. A person, thus, could be classified as being "blind" if he/she had a significant vision loss, but he/she would not necessarily share such attributes as spatially disoriented or be awkward in walking. A disjunctive concept has the advantage that it permits the creation of many subgroups in which specific and significant attributes form the basis for an intervention strategy. It has the disadvantage of making it all but impossible to find meaningful groups in a small population such as the blind. In fact, it leads to the very difficult situation in which each individual is seen as being unique. That, in turn, would mean that expensive, albeit highly effective, service programs would be needed to assist in maximizing development of children or clients. While this is the expressed ideal for special education and rehabilitation, that ideal has not been achieved due to the conjunctive concepts currently in vogue. Just as with the need to create a legal definition of blindness, current needs for classifications have the effect of limiting costs rather than helping all children and clients meet their potential.

The logical conclusion to the use of disjunctive concepts would be to all but eliminate the need for a taxonomy for such broad groupings as "blindness," "deafness," "mental retardation," and other such groupings, and it would further require professionals to provide services with a flexible approach. It would require great amounts of creativity and ingenuity. This in turn, would cost more money and would not appear at all to be economical or, it might allow unique individuals to develop to the point that they could be far more productive than those enclosed within a broader and flatter category.

TWENTY QUESTIONS

As discussed in earlier sections, generic descriptions do not identify unique characteristics of individuals. More specific phenotype or genotype characteristics are needed to begin to identify, describe, and remember the vast array of plants, animals, and minerals that make up the world in which people live. It may be even more difficult to describe, classify, and remember complex concepts in the nonmaterial domain of thought. Efficient cognitive strategies for remembering are important to success in everyday life. As discussed above, categorization is helpful in memory and retrieval of information. Categories also help define relationships and common attributes so that through the use of key concepts or words, the professional can make decisions quickly. Those who are unable to categorize are very likely to have difficulty identifying, describing, and remembering, reading, and more importantly, understanding what is read as well as other forms of categorizing that are essential to learning either academic content or routine tasks needed each day.

It is quite probable that like any other characteristic, the abilities to categorize, see relationships, and recall can be placed on a continuum between not able to perform to best performance. Perhaps even more important these abilities can most likely be improved through experience and practice. An example of practice is the game of 20 questions.

The object of the game is to identify the specific item submitted by an audience by asking no more than 20 questions. A moderator simply states whether the object is animal, vegetable, or mineral or part vegetable, and part mineral. Team members then ask questions which could be answered yes or no. By asking questions that eliminated large categories the object can often be identified within the questions asked. For example a question that might be asked about an animal might be: Does the animal live on land? Of course, if the answer was "no," the team could be sure that a guess of camel would not be correct. So the next question might be: "Is it a mammal?" If the answer was "yes," then all fishes would be eliminated as possible answers, and so on. Another example you might like to try is to determine how many questions it takes to locate a square located within a figure made of 10 squares across and 10 squares down, 100 squares in all. Suppose a friend thinks of a number from 1 to 100, such as 83, and that the squares are numbered as shown in the example below. How many questions will be needed to identify the unknown number?

1	2	3	4	5	6	7	8	9	10
11	12	13	14	15	16	17	18	19	20
21	22	23	24	25	26	27	28	29	30
31	32	33	34	35	36	37	38	39	40
41	42	43	44	45	46	47	48	49	50
51	52	53	54	55	56	57	58	59	60
61	62	63	64	65	66	67	68	69	70
71	72	73	74	75	76	77	78	79	80
81	82	83	84	85	86	87	88	89	90
91	92	93	94	95	96	97	98	99	**100**

Figure 2.1. There is an equal chance of selecting the right number with the first try as after 100 tries. Those who do not have strategies for categorizing have difficulty learning either academic content or routine tasks needed each day. Problem solving becomes random with little chance of immediate success.

The first strategy might be to simply guess at random. "Is it 19? Is it 55? Is ...." While the questioner might be correct on the first guess it is also possible that it would take 100 guesses to find the correct square. This may be an approach used by a small child who sees no sequence or cannot, because of lack of experience with number relationship, know of another strategy.

The randomness, unless the person guessing had high rewards for correct answers, or guessed correctly often enough to make the game fun, would soon discourage the player. However, in real life, individuals do not always have the choice of not playing but are forced to keep guessing because there is not an infinite number of things and strategies for categorizing available.

A second approach might be based on the numbers themselves. For example, one might ask the following, "Is it an even number? No. Is it a number above 25? No. Is it a number below 9? Yes," and so forth. Here the questions have been much more efficient requiring a maximum of seven questions.

1	2	3	4	5	6	7	8	9	10
11	12	13	14	15	16	17	18	19	20
21	22	23	24	25	26	27	28	29	30
31	32	33	34	35	36	37	38	39	40
41	42	43	44	45	46	47	48	49	50
51	52	53	54	55	56	57	58	59	60
61	62	63	64	65	66	67	68	69	70
71	72	73	74	75	76	77	78	79	80
81	82	83	84	85	86	87	88	89	90
91	92	93	94	95	96	97	98	99	100

Figure 2.2. Categories themselves, such as even numbers or other classifications, reduce random guessing and help in decision making.

1	2	3	4	5	6	7	8	9	10
11	12	13	14	15	16	17	18	19	20
21	22	23	24	25	26	27	28	29	30
31	32	33	34	35	36	37	38	39	40
41	42	43	44	45	46	47	48	49	50
51	52	53	54	55	56	57	58	59	60
61	62	63	64	65	66	67	68	69	70
71	72	73	74	75	76	77	78	79	80
81	82	83	84	85	86	87	88	89	90
91	92	93	94	95	96	97	98	99	100

Figure 2.3. Understanding categories related to locations and spatial relationships provides another strategy for selecting solutions to problems encountered each day.

Still another strategy might be to search by location in the square. The questions might be, "Is it in the top half? No. Is it left of center? Yes. Is it in the top half of the lower quadrant? No. Is it left of center in the lower quadrant? No. Is it on the bottom row? No," and so on. One might wonder if these strategies are effected by sensory loss and if so, how are these strategies effected by sensory loss.

Most individuals will have abilities to employ these strategies to a greater or lesser degree. The major factors which determine an individual's ability are genotypic characteristics such as heredity, experiences which create a need and allow for categorization and phenotypic characteristics such as blindness, deafness, orthopedic impairments, etc. The latter two are of concern here since until genetic engineering is better developed heredity will be predetermined at birth.

What about those who are not normal, whether from lack of experience or because of some other observable characteristic such as a disability? Special methods have been designed to remediate the experience deficits, as in the case when English needs to be taught as a second language. Likewise, overcoming vision loss requires strategies different from general education, but there is a difference which must be addressed. The difference is a disability. To be more specific, no amount of training, goal setting, or physical adaptation will make the person see. The result is the same as if the genotype had been changed. Of course, the effect on the individual will depend on the degree of the disabling problem and when the disability occurred. Some effect will result which requires changes in the experiences meant to educate if the person is to achieve normal expectations and overcome the handicap.

For most individuals, a generic picture of development, such as a developmental scale or a standardized achievement test is adequate for describing the level of ability. When gaps are identified in what is considered normal for the general population, then general solutions can be suggested to meet the needs of the general population. Public education is one of the best examples of this approach. A need was identified for the general population to be literate, to be trained in habits that support the industrial revolution and the society which it created and to perpetuate the national political systems. The education system designed to meet these needs in the United States has worked well for over two centuries. Recently, the change from the industrial age to the information age has made it necessary to reevaluate the needs and perhaps to design new strategies of education to meet the general (generic) needs of the population.

There is, and seemingly always has been, uncertainty about how to provide equal opportunities for those who have visual disabilities. The debate usually has been based on beliefs concerning the status of individuals who are blind rather than recognizing the unique effects of vision loss on the individual's altered cognitive abilities which are due to the absence of sight.

Except in rare instances, usually associated with retinal blastoma, those born without sight have difficulties with spatial concepts. The experiences that develop spatial categories usually come through the sense of sight. When a visual disability is present from birth, normal development cannot occur. The lack of visual input can be shown to effect the structure and size of the brain in laboratory animals and presumably has similar effects in humans. Lack of development of visual areas of the brain certainly affects the ability to categorize, and recall visual experiences related to spatial concepts. This, in turn, affects such things as understanding the visual characteristics of objects, figure-ground relationships, as well as distance and time relationships. When these areas are affected, the ability to orient in space and travel independently must be developed by special, alternative methods. The field of peripetology (orientation and mobility) is one of the disciplines which goes far beyond the general educator's expertise and is an example of why separate categories of teacher preparation, and instructional systems are necessary for those with visual disabilities.

It could be concluded that since there is an inherent deficit that it is useless to attempt to help individuals who are blind become normal. Indeed, some in the public often take a very paternalistic view of services which should be provided because their expectations are so low. The fact that thousands of blind persons who have had special training which provided concepts via alternative sensory experiences, assistive technologies, and specific teaching methods are independent, caring, and responsible citizens clearly demonstrates that efforts to overcome the deficits are successful. Further, special programs are valuable both to the individual and to the general society.

If it is true that special knowledge and methods are needed for all individuals to be able to acquire cognitive strategies for survival and success in life; and if programs which can provide alternative methods for achieving the same goals for disabled individuals are available;

then society has also become the beneficiary and should continue to be supportive of these approaches. Educators and policymakers do not seem to question the value of attempting alternative ways for assisting individuals with disabilities to achieve the same goals at the same levels as those without disabilities. The only question is whether power can be applied to accomplish the task with generalists, or is it better to provide special services to individuals based on groups or categories.

Perhaps a way to decide whether a separate discipline is needed in work for the blind is to discover whether the impact of sight loss affects enough ability domains to warrant a categorically based system to meet the needs. Descriptions of the impact of blindness will be presented in later chapters.

ORGANIZATIONS FOR AND OF THE BLIND

Thus far, there has been a discussion of whether it is beneficial to have categories of disabilities. Among the blind, the existence of this same issue can be demonstrated. Some organizations attempt to serve all interests of the blind. These include such organizations as the Affiliated Leadership League of and for the Blind (ALL), American Council of the Blind (ACB), National Federation of the Blind (NFB), National Association of Parents of the Visually Impaired (NAPVI) and Association for Education and Rehabilitation of the Blind and Visually Impaired (AER). Reason for these inclusive organizations within the blind community is that often the needs of the blind lack sufficient numbers to advocate for very specific needs when addressed by only those who have the specific need. To Illustrate, each of the large groups of adult blind, the ACB and the NFB, as well as the professional organization, AER, has chapters and divisions which meet very specific needs such as those who use dog guides, those who are blind lawyers, those who teach preschool, those who have low vision, those who have. . . . The list of special interests within the community of the blind is very lengthy.

Each of the special interest groups performs a service for the blind or is composed of individuals who are blind. Usually the name of the organization tells whether the members of the group are blind or serve the blind. However, the title does not exclude either function. A group of blind persons might also serve the blind. For example, members of the blind ham radio group has as its purpose to assist blind persons with materials to help pass the amateur radio exam.

In addition to the stated purpose of the organization or common reasons for affiliation, there are philosophical issues associated with the terms of and for. The crux of the philosophical argument is whether blind individuals can speak for themselves or not. Even then, one will have to look at how the organization functions to determine which philosophy the group espouses. Each group obviously meets some need of some group of people. The diverse needs call for diverse ways of meeting the needs. So, again, it can be seen that categorical services are more powerful in meeting the needs of individuals. Resistance to categories are generated in efforts to economize the use of resources or make services uniform for all participants. These restraints make services less powerful for the individual.

Though there is diversity among organizations of and for the blind, the authors believe there is strong consensus that all of them feel that categorical services that meet the needs of the blind rather than generic services for all disability groups provide a better means of serving blind persons. This sometimes is viewed by other groups as the blind being unwilling to collaborate. The authors further believe that the sentiment for categorical services comes from experiences with generic agencies which have reduced services to the blind and that these organizations have a great deal to offer and are willing to support many generic issues related to social, political, and funding concerns. As mentioned earlier, there are a large number of organizations that specifically relate to work for the blind, too many to present here.

DISCUSSION

This chapter deals with the idea that the world is extremely complex. For example, it has been suggested that the normal human eye can distinguish or discriminate about seven-and-a-half million different colors, yet people have a color vocabulary of a couple of dozen names. Humans categorize in order to simplify the world. If people were to subdivide all categories to their logical conclusions, they would still have the same level of complexity as before the process started since everything is unique when examined in terms of a complete listing of attributes.

If oversimplification is used, power is lost, everything becomes vague and no meaningful distinctions can be made. If categorization is done too completely, the simplification is lost. Obviously, there is a need to make some categories more complete in areas which are of most interest, and to use broader categories for areas where there is little interest. Some areas may not need categories at all, e.g., in areas where no knowledge at all is needed.

Recent movements in special education, probably for administrators' convenience and as an economy move, have tended to eliminate higher-order categories based on etiologies of educational difficulties. It has been claimed that knowing the cause of a difficulty does not lead to specific remediations for all persons in specific categories such as vision or hearing loss. Rather, it is claimed that regular education can use traditional methods, supplemented with assistance from specialists, to solve most of the problems.

In this and subsequent chapters, the authors demonstrate their belief that the categorical approach is the most useful, cost effective, and productive approach for the education and rehabilitation of persons with vision losses. That does not mean that all of the problems have been solved, but at present, there are no alternative methods which have demonstrated better results based on hard, empirical research data.

SUGGESTED READINGS

1. Stevens, G.D. (1962). *Taxonomy in special education for children with body disorder: The problem and a proposal.* Doctoral Dissertation. Columbia University, New York, NY.

Chapter 3

GROWTH AND DEVELOPMENT

INTRODUCTION

"Disabled children are more like nondisabled children than they are different." University level, special education students are taught this and later teach the same. While the statement is true, it is essentially meaningless for professionals working with exceptional children where the "differences" must be identified and remediated. The statement is based on the use of "quiet" attributes which are shared by almost all living things. Thus, flies are more like elephants than they are different since they both eat, move, take in oxygen, reproduce their kind, die, and so on. One cannot assist children with visual impairments unless the nature of the impairments, disabilities, and/or handicaps are clearly in focus and skills available to provide appropriate assistance.

In this chapter, the authors will focus on some aspects of growth and development which are shared by all children and then consider other factors which are common to children with vision problems. The discussion of the development of "normal" children will not be exhaustive since other sources are available with that focus.

The child with vision problems, like normally seeing children, goes through stages which take the child from infancy to adulthood. Growth refers to the genetically controlled processes which govern physical maturation and biological unfolding. Development refers to the social and environmental processes which surround the growing child and which interact with the genetic makeup to form a living human organism in a cultural setting. Geneticists have discovered sufficient diversity in the human genome to account for the tremendous diversity in human beings; likewise, developmental psychologists and social scientists have described sufficient diversity in the social and environmental milieu to account for the same human diversity. Most professionals in human services accept elements from both developmental and behavioral approaches to explain how children grow to become adults.

Growth and development describe the processes by which the newborn infant becomes a productive and participating member of a society. This process is usually divided into several areas such as motor, psychosocial, and cognitive development. These, in turn, can be further subdivided into more specific skills such as walking, speaking, or problem solving.

In this chapter, the authors will confine themselves to the two broad areas of motor and psychosocial growth and development, with cognitive and emotional development the topic of another chapter.

Once a general background in growth and development is established, it will be beneficial to compare persons with visual handicaps with their sighted peers. Where differences are noted, methods must be applied which will allow for maximizing the developmental potential of persons with visual disabilities and handicaps.

OBJECTIVES

At the completion of this chapter readers should be able to;

1. Describe the principles which guide the understanding of normal motor development.
2. Identify the leading figures in the study of motor development and psychological research.
3. Define, compare, and contrast four theories of psychosocial development.
4. Demonstrate an understanding of the differences in psychosocial development of persons with visual handicaps in contrast to persons with normal sight.
5. Suggest areas in which additional research is needed in order to better understand the growth and development of persons with visual handicaps.
6. Identify and describe several remedial approaches which can be used with various age groups of children with visual handicaps.

SCIENCE OF GROWTH AND DEVELOPMENT

The scientific study of growth and development involves the careful, orderly, and systematic observations of changes in the patterns of children's' actions and appearances. It is generally assumed that this process begins with the "zygote" or the fertilized ovum. The human zygote contains 23 pairs of chromosomes, one of the pairs from the father and one from the mother. These are made of atoms and molecules of proteins and sugars in a form described as a "spiral staircases" with the proteins making up the handrails and the sections of sugars and other elements forming the "rungs." Combinations of these "sections" constitute "genes." Guided by a timed order, genes are expressed by producing changes in the structures and functions of cells in the body. The expression of genes takes place in a context of factors and forces which influence that expression. The 23 pairs of chromosomes with their gene segments constitute the "blueprint" of the body. This "blueprint" is housed in the nucleus of every cell in the body. The genetic material is referred to as "deoxyribonucleic acid" or "DNA." Various enzymes interact with the strands of DNA to permit the use of specific parts of the strand for growth of specific parts of the body at the appropriate time. The information in the DNA is coded by combinations of four amino acid nucleotide, or peptides, or protein molecules. These nucleotide (adenine, thymine, cytosine, and guanine) are located at the same places on each of the two strands of DNA which are inherited from the father and the mother and represent the points where the "ladder's rungs" join. As an enzyme opens up a segment of the spiral staircase, a duplicate of one of the strands is made from Ribonucleic Acid (RNA) with the exception that uracil, another nucleotide, is substituted for thymine. This "messenger RNA" carries the information to the cytoplasm or fluid which surrounds the cell nucleus and there additional copies of the RNA are formed to make specific parts of the cell's membrane wall or other parts of the cell.

Processes have recently been discovered which monitor the structure of the DNA and make corrections when an error is found. This process is not foolproof, however, since genetic defects and cancers still occur.

Five general growth patterns have emerged from the application of scientific methodology. These are:

1. Differentiation: This involves changes from the global toward the specific, from the simple toward the complex, from the homogeneous toward the heterogeneous, and from the general toward the specific.
2. Hierarchal Integration: Structures and functions become organized into interconnected levels.
3. Discontinuous Growth: Change does not occur in a smooth, continuous fashion, but as rapid spurts followed by plateaus.
4. Growth Discontinuity: Growth occurs in spurts and starts with periods of no change followed by rapid change.
5. Growth Gradients: Growth starts at the head and moves toward the tail–cephalo-caudal–and from the inside out–proximo-distal.

It is generally understood that these growth patterns occur within a single individual, but exactly when do the patterns begin? At the time of birth, or at the time of conception, or back through many generations of ancestors? It is most likely the latter, but the description usually begins with conception.

For the first two months after conception, the individual is referred to as an "embryo." During this period the zygote begins the process of cell division, with no differences noted between the "mother" and "daughter" cells. The first differentiation occurs with the cells at the top of the embryo. This change is in the form of neurons or nerve cells which form the neural cap and is the beginning of the nervous system. These gray cells begin to thicken, then to form a groove. The groove becomes the spinal column and the cranium neural cap becomes the brain. Near the end of the embryonic period, two frontal extensions of the neural cap emerge which will become the optic nerves and retinas of the eyes.

After the differentiation of neurons or nerve cells begins, other differentiations occur which result in the development of the internal organs, bones, and muscles of the body. The various parts do not grow at the same rate and the growth does not proceed smoothly. For example, until recently it has been believed that the nervous system has all of the nerve cells it will ever have by the end of the first six months of prenatal growth when the individual is referred to as the "fetus." New studies appear to show that some neurons are created in the brain even until very late in life. The patterns of neural growth seem to follow specific patterns. Perhaps this "priority" development indicates the importance of the nervous system for the individual.

All of the growth patterns are illustrated in the growth of the nervous system during this prenatal period, but they will be repeated in the growth that occurs after birth in the newborn child. The nervous system–cephalo–is the first system to begin and is the first completed. It also begins with the structures of the internal nervous system–proximo–followed by more distal elements such as the retinas of the eyes.

MOTOR DEVELOPMENT

The newborn infant is extremely uncoordinated, with arms and legs, head and trunk moving in essentially random patterns. But as time passes, the child first learns to move the eyes, then the head and neck, through the arms and onto the legs. Control is at first very limited. In their first months of life, the child begins to coordinate general movements of the several parts of the body and the limbs. Crawling, creeping, sitting, standing, walking, etc. all move from more global toward more specific actions with ever-increasing control over movements.

In the meantime, the internal body organs have been maturing and controlling digestion, heart actions, temperature control, etc. Few of the internal growth and metabolic processes are fully matured, however, until long after the end of childhood, including both fine motor and gross motor functions.

Studies have revealed that maturation–an unfolding of innate potentials–is largely in control of the inborn patterns. For example, training one of a set of identical twins to ride a tricycle several months before the other does not result in an advantage for the earlier-trained over the later-trained twin in tricycle riding ability. The person develops motor skills when the time is right. Vocalization skills follow a similar sequential pattern of development. It is not until later childhood and adolescence that practice in motor skills produces improvements of performance over mere unfoldment.

PSYCHOSOCIAL DEVELOPMENT

Since psychosocial development typically is observed in relationship to persons, events, and objects outside and beyond the individual, the developmental patterns are not so obvious nor as dependent on genetic unfolding. Nevertheless, the patterns appear to follow the same common sequences. The various theories described in the developmental literature indicate, however, that different theorists have chosen different aspects of development to reflect these patterns. Most of these theories have leaned heavily on Sigmond Freud's work. However, Freud's observations were based on analysis of adults who came to him for maladaptive behavior. It would seem that such observations would provide inappropriate data from which to make appropriate generalizations to child development and particularly to development of children with impaired sight. It seems to the authors that, if the foundations upon which these theories are built is faulty, the superstructure will not be very accurate or useful. The impact of faulty theories of psychological development may create greater harm for those with visual impairments than for those who grew up with normal visual abilities.

The rest of this section on psychosocial development will give a brief overview of some of the leading theorist's beliefs. Each one has a contribution to make and those interested in working with children who are blind or have low vision should be careful to understand how each relates to the development of children.

Freud

As alluded to above, Freud was perhaps the first to consider child development from a psychological perspective. His major contributions were the ideas that development occurs in stages and that reasons for behavior could be identified through careful observations and analysis of the person's history. He, like those who later studied child development, provided general ages when major changes in development occur and described those stages.

Freud described three influences on development the id, the ego, and the superego. The interaction of these three allowed for identification of stages as the child grew. The ages are very general and include the following:

1. The Anal Stage: successful feeding and use of the mouth as a means of information and gratification.

2. Toilet training and the resulting conflicts regarding compliance and external demands.
3. The Phallic Stage: Body awareness, gender identity and role development.
4. The Latency Stage: Repression of sexual issues and development of childhood tasks.
5. Genital Stage: Development of a mature personality and development of intimate relationships.

These stages occur from birth to adolescence and in the sequence listed. Development is considered maladaptive when the stages are out of sequence or when they persist too long.

Eric Erickson

Erickson is viewed as a Neo-Freudian. His beliefs center more on social influences rather than biological issues. Erickson's beliefs were gained from his studies of various cultures and settings. His theories of social development center around each individual's quest for a separate identity stated in terms of the conflicts that occur in reaching independence. The stages are:

1. Trust vs. Mistrust
2. Autonomy vs. Shame/Doubt
3. Initiative vs. Guilt
4. Industry vs. Inferiority
5. Identity vs. Role Diffusion

Erickson also considered that there is a sequence of stages. The major difference in Erickson's theory is that each stage of development is the result of factors found within a culture. The optimal setting would foster trust, autonomy, initiative, industry, and self-identity rather than mistrust, shame, guild, inferiority, and role diffusion.

R. J. Havighurst

Perhaps being influenced by both Freud and Erickson, Havighurst combined the notions of biological and social affects on the development of individuals. The stages he describes, as noted in Scholl (1986) are as follows:

Stage 1. Learning to take solid foods, learning to walk, learning to talk.

Stage 2. Learning to control the elimination of bodily wastes, learning sex differences and sexual modesty, forming concepts and learning language to describe social and physical reality, getting ready to read.

Stage 3. Learning physical skills for ordinary games; building wholesome attitudes towards oneself as a growing organism; learning to get along with age-mates; learning an appropriate masculine or feminine role; developing fundamental skills in reading, writing, and calculating; developing concepts necessary for everyday living; developing conscience, morality, and a scale of values; achieving personal independence; developing attitudes toward social groups and institutions.

Stage 4. Achieving new and more mature relations with age-mates, achieving a masculine or feminine social role, accepting one's physique and using body effectively, achieving emotional independence of parents and other adults, preparing for marriage and family life, preparing for economic career, acquiring a set of values and an ethical system as a guide to behavior, desiring and achieving socially responsible behavior.

The complexity of psychosocial development becomes evident when trying to understand Havighurst's use of the previous ideas described by Freud and Erickson. Each stage is described in more detail; however, there are many more tasks for educators when helping children to achieve these tasks.

Kohlberg

Kohlberg moves farther from the impact of physical growth than Freud, Erickson, and Havighurst. His theory relates to moral development. His theory describes four stages of moral development with two parts for each. In brief, the stages and parts are as follows.

1. Completely egocentric: No moral concepts, fear of punishment
2. Preconventional: Punishment and obedience orientation, instrumental relativist orientation

3. Conventional: Interpersonal concordance orientation, society systems and conscience maintenance
4. Postconventional: Social contract orientation, universal ethical principle orientation.

This theory seems to move away from external causes of psychosocial development toward an internal orientation. In other words, the psychosocial development is more a function of cognitive learning than behavior caused by biological or cultural influences. This would seem to match the stages of cognitive development described by Jean Piaget.

Piaget's theories of cognitive development will be discussed in a later chapter. As will also be seen in a later chapter, studies of cognitive development have been more rigorous and avoided some problems of inadequate and inappropriate models on which to base theory and practices and have provided far more useful constructs. Perhaps the psychosocial developmental theorists need to go back to the drawing board and begin from the premises which have guided other research on aspects of growth and development.

GROWTH AND DEVELOPMENT IN CHILDREN
WITH VISUAL IMPAIRMENTS

In the previous sections, normal physical growth and development, as well as some theories of psychosocial development, have been described. However, the ways in which lack of vision impacts these processes has not been adequately demonstrated. The lack of information about how blind children and adults are affected by vision loss is because the diversity of this low incident blind population does not provide easily reachable homogeneous groups for study.

In spite of the lack of an extensive body of formal research, it is clear that lack of sight impacts development in many ways. What is less certain is whether adjustments to the physical and social environments can overcome the disabilities created by sight loss. David Warren (1984) addresses the need for much more study. There are many examples which describe difference in development between blind and sighted children. These include delays in motor development, difference in language development interruptions, or delays in social development and differences in cognitive reasoning. Only a few will be discussed here to illustrate and cause consideration of the differences observed.

For the most part, both motor and psychosocial development in children with visual handicaps follow the same patterns as those for children with normal sight. There are some differences, however, which should be taken note of. For example, as noted in the research literature, infants with no sight do not seem to like being in the prone position, i.e., being on their stomachs (Hart 1974). This seems to result in slower development of such motor skills as crawling and walking. There is considerable evidence that delayed development of motor skills and the consequent reduction of incoming stimulation from the environment sometimes result in the acquisition of "blindisms" or stereotyped, self-stimulation behaviors. Perhaps the absence of sight means that the child is not motivated to move toward objects.

The same lack of sight limits the ability of the child with no sight to interact with adults around him/her. A normal child is programmed to look at a caregiver's eyes, making a social contact that promotes bonding. Lack of sight interferes with bonding to parent simply because eye contact is not important to the blind infant and lack of eye contact may discourage the normal interactions of the parent.

Further, as the child without sight grows and is more aware of the environment, his/her methods of gaining information may discourage interactions. To illustrate, when a child with sight sees an adult, he or she may become more animated, waving arms and legs, and smiling which encourages the parent to pay attention and pick the child up. In contrast, the blind child may hear movement and quiet to gain more information by listening and, if suddenly lifted, become disoriented or frightened and cry. A parent who does not recognize the cause of the child's crying behavior can soon become conditioned to believe the child is happier when left alone. Thus, social interaction needed for bonding and learning are reduced and cause slower development of socialization.

Still later social relationships with peers are also affected by lack of sight. When a child or an adult is unable to see, it is difficult to compete especially in unstructured ways. As an example, without a structured routine for daily tasks, such as brushing teeth, doing laundry, and traveling, it takes more time than normal to accomplish tasks if the blind person has to search by feeling rather than scanning visually for items not close at hand. The slowing down or alternative way of accomplishing many common tasks creates some real and some imagined "handicaps." Differences in development because of lack of sight put the child with no sight at a disadvantage in later competition with seeing age mates.

It must be stressed that even though many description of blind children indicate significant delays in major developmental domains, the causes are not clear. Blind people are successful in all areas of life and have become physically normal and have accommodated to the social environment. Perhaps different abilities may be necessary in order to accomplish the same tasks at a competitive level with those who see normally. However, differences in methods should not imply inferiority.

The book by David Warren, *Blindness and Early Childhood Development* (1984), is recommended as the best summary of available research on the development of children with visual handicaps and the implications of such development in later life. It is not easy reading for the neophyte in this field, but it constitutes a very valuable resource for the professional worker in this discipline of blindness. A careful reading of that book will provide some of the more useful findings in this area and provide suggestions for remediating deficits in developmental patterns in children with visual impairments. By using one's imagination and creativity, other ideas for remediation should become apparent.

DISCUSSION

This chapter has attempted to lay a foundation for readers' understanding of the motor and social development of children with visual impairments. It also should point you toward other areas of growth and development which need to be studied. It has *not* dealt with all aspects of these topics and it should be explicitly understood that the reader will need to continue to study the problems in development which are related to vision loss. A single human brain is more complex than any other phenomenon with which scientists are acquainted. It is more complex even than the known universe in that it is able to understand virtually anything in that universe except, perhaps, itself. With this idea ever present before the reader, he/she should be able to avoid the problem of becoming "an expert" in child development with final answers to all remaining questions.

SUGGESTED READINGS

1. Scholl, G.T. (1986). *Foundations of education for blind and visually handicapped children and youth: Theory and practice.* New York: American Foundation for the Blind.
2. Warren, D. (1984). *Blindness and early childhood development.* New York: American Foundation for the Blind.
3. Hart, V. (1974). *Beginning with the handicapped.* Springfield, IL: Charles C Thomas.

Chapter 4

COGNITIVE DEVELOPMENT

INTRODUCTION

That which most contrasts people with other living creatures is their intellectual ability. Although apes have been taught to communicate with sign language, there is no evidence that they pass this ability on to their offspring, and their offspring must learn sign language in the same fashion as their parents, e.g., by being taught by human beings.

Ernest Seeton Thompson, the great naturalist of a generation ago, observed that there are three levels of communication among living things: reflexive communication, in which there is no seeming intention to communicate; intentional communication, in which one creature intends to influence another by movements or sounds; and syntactical communication in which information is abstracted and communicated through use of specific and agreed-upon rules. An example of reflexive communication is the information given by honey bees when they return to the hive after foraging, in which the number of turns of the body and the angle of elevation of the body during a dance gives information to other bees. Intentional communication is illustrated by the dog barking to warn a child of a nearby danger. Syntactical communication is illustrated by human communication. There is some evidence that porpoises communicate with one another, but it is highly unlikely that this communication involves syntactical communication. In fact, scientists have not found clear evidence of syntactical communication in any other form of life.This chapter, which shows that children with visual handicaps do not markedly differ from children with sight, shows that they can communicate and perform other intellectual tasks as effectively as children with normal sight. They may not demonstrate their intellectual skills in exactly the same manner as others, yet they are still not intellectually retarded as a consequence of vision loss. This suggests that the teacher can and should expect fairly normal performance from children with visual handicaps in areas of life where intelligence is important.

As noted in Chapter 1, much of what is learned about our environments (both external and internal) results from sensory experiences. There are other factors involved, however, since all children seem to move through very similar sequences of development. This would suggest that some general innate or genetic process guides this development. The content of each person's "world view" may differ, but the sequences are very similar. This is clearly the case in motor development. In psychosocial development, the stages are not so nearly well recognized. Not only does content vary from person to person and culture to culture, but the stages are not clearly evident. Jean Piaget has provided a description of stages of cognitive development which are observable in children world wide. Cultural environments guide progress through these stages, providing the experiences which foster or retard progress, but the stages appear to be invariant. Piaget illustrates these stages of development with examples drawn from the western culture, especially with Swiss children. If the reader is familiar with development in other cultures such as American Indian, he/she may wish to see if one can observe similar patterns in children from that culture.

Hebb and Thompson argue, and illustrate their argument from research data, that cognitive and emotional development are interactive or even, perhaps, the same. Children have inborn tendencies to react emotionally to different environments. These reactions emerge and differentiate as the child grows, and that cultural environment structures how emotions can be properly expressed. For example, violence is emotionally arousing in all cultures and in all individuals. But, each culture has developed its own mores, manners, standards, etc. which guide the expression of the emotions. One culture might punish actions aroused by emotions with restraint or imprisonment, while another might exploit such reactivity by placing the individual into a military unit. The actions and sounds of eating are also emotionally arousing, but one culture may consider "burping" a compliment to the cook while another will ostracize the "noisy" eater. Hebb and Thompson also illustrate their theory by citing examples from the animal world which demonstrate changes in both cognitive and affective development. Rats, lower than dogs on the Phyletic Scale, are less intelligent and less emotionally reactive. Dogs, lower on the phyletic scale than chimpanzees but higher than rats, show fewer emotions than "chimps," but more than rats and, at the same time, are "smarter" than rats but less intelligent than chimps.

If, as noted above, environments guide the expression of genetically produced action tendencies, then children with visual impairments should have the same genetic tendencies as other children, both in terms of cognitive and affective development, but would have a different environment in which these tendencies are expressed. This is because the information from the external environment in particular will have major gaps in specific knowledge. Thus, the stages of development, which appear to be under genetic control, would differ for children with visual impairments in much the same way children from different cultures differ from one another.

Research supports the belief that children with no sight do not differ from children with sight in intelligence. Where deficits do appear—as for example in spatial awareness—the difference is probably related to an information gap and not from a genetic deficit. It would seem that cognitive development is mediated by language skills. As noted in Chapter 2 of this text, people use language to encode and label concepts. Language also provides the framework for interrelating and structuring concepts. An analysis of the game "20 Questions" shows that most people organize concepts in an hierarchy, with broader, more general concepts superordinate to small, more specific concepts.

Since children with visual impairments seem to organize their conceptual world in terms of language and, therefore, seem to have few deficits, this language hierarchical "program" seems to be innate. In the case of children with hearing impairments, language does not develop normally, and so their academic development is much slower. This would strongly suggest that auditory information, especially language, is the indispensable key to maximum cognitive and language development. For example, Helen Keller's cognitive development moved ahead very rapidly once she realized that words could be used to represent objects.

In Chapter 3, the authors began a discussion of a child's growth and development with theories of motor and psychosocial development.

This chapter will continue with theories of cognitive and affective or emotional development. The major foci of the chapter will be on how children gain knowledge about their environments (both external and internal), how emotions develop, and the way in which cognitive and emotional development interact.

OBJECTIVES

At the completion of this chapter the reader should be able to:

1. Describe and cite examples of the four major stages of cognitive development as posited by Jean Piaget together with a demonstration of an awareness of the six substages for sensory-motor and the two substages of the preoperational stage.
2. Understand the process Piaget followed in developing his theory.
3. Identify the relationship between cognitive development as described by Hebb and Thompson.
4. Discuss in a coherent manner what effects cognitive and affective development result from vision loss, and how these effects might be remediated with appropriate interventions.

JEAN PIAGET'S THEORY OF INTELLECT

The "hallmark" of Piaget's method for assessing a child's concept of "conservation" is two clay or play dough balls, about two inches in diameter. Obtain two such balls. Select two children of different ages. Work with them separately so one will not influence the other's responses.Present to the child the two balls and ask, "Are these balls the SAME, or are they DIFFERENT?" If the child agrees that they are the same, proceed. If the child says they are different, ask him/her to make them the same. When the child is satisfied, proceed.Now, take one of the balls and roll it into the shape of a "hot dog." Then ask the child, "Is there still the same amount of clay in the ball and the hot dog, or is there more clay in the hot dog or the ball?"

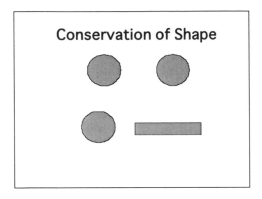

Figure 4.1. Conservation of shape. Genetic unfoldment interacts with environmental pressures to produce mental structures which allow the child to understand that a shape does not change the amount of clay.

Write or record what the child says. Ask, "How do you know?" Again, note what the child says. Next, roll the hot dog back into a ball, and ask the same question as before. Note answers. Next, mold one of the balls into a pancake shape. Repeat the question as before. Note answers and ask "Why is that?" or "How do you know?" Repeat this same experiment with the second child. Typically, Piaget has found children below the age of six or seven years will view the ball with the modified shape as possessing more clay. They will not recognize that the shape of a ball does not change its volume or mass. Piaget described in his theory dynamic processes which guide the development of intelligence. Changes occur when the present intellectual structures—"schemas"—are inadequate for a person to solve problems of coping with the environment. If the child's present levels of genetic development are appropriate, then new schemas will emerge which will enhance problem solutions. This is a continuous process. Genetic unfoldment interacts with environmental pressures to produce mental structures which allow the child to cope more and more effectively with perceived problems of living. A dynamic balance—"equilibration"—is constantly being established and then upset and then reestablished. Piaget's major contribution is this description of the processes of cognitive development and the structures which emerge.

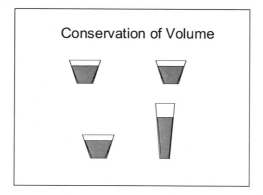

Figure 4.2. Conservation of volume. The shape of the glass does not change the amount of water.

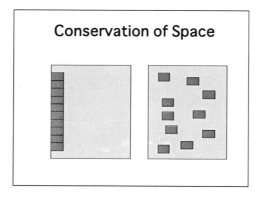

Figure 4.3. Conservation of space. Location of equal size and number of objects does not change the size of an area.

FACTORS OF INTELLIGENCE

David Wechsler, author of the Wechsler tests of intelligence, defined intelligence as: The global or aggregate capacity of the individual to think rationally, act purposefully and to deal effectively with the environment. Lewis Terman, the author of the Stanford-Binet Intelligence Scales, defines intelligence as: The possession of a large number of clearly-defined concepts, the ability to see coherent and meaningful interrelationships among these concepts, and to apply these concepts in the solution of problems. While there are other definitions, these underlie much of present-day psychology. The Wechsler and Terman tests are the most widely used measures of intelligence in English-speaking countries throughout the world. J. P. Guilford, in his article, "The Three Faces of Intellect," provides a structural analysis of intelligence in terms of the three dimensions of content or input, operations or processes, and products or outputs. By looking at the subdivisions of these three dimensions, it is possible to notice the existence of about 120 separate intellective factors. These factors describe the wide variations in performances of every-day actions. These definitions and descriptions represent a static, point-in-time picture of intelligence rather than how the elements develop and change dynamically.

Even with these definitions and descriptions, the nature of intelligence is not agreed upon. There is one camp which holds that intelligence is a general or "G" factor which underlies the ability to cope with all aspects of life. There is another camp which claims that there are many specific factors of intelligence—"aptitudes"—which are specific to the accomplishment of specific kinds of tasks. Terman, for example, saw intelligence as a generalized ability to solve widely differing problems. Guilford, on the other hand, saw intelligence as a large number of narrower, more specific skills or abilities related to fewer task solutions. Raymond B. Cattell, in 1962, conducted statistical analyses of test results and suggested that intelligence can be reduced to two types of intellective factors: "crystallized intelligence," which is essentially structures of learned problem solutions; and "fluid intelligence," which is essentially the process used by an individual as new problems are solved. Most intelligence tests, he claims, measure crystallized intelligence.

Biologists distinguish between two types of characteristics of living things: "phenotypic" characteristics, which are observable, surface properties; and "genotypic" properties which are unobserved, underlying factors based on genetic structures and processes which find expression in different phenotypic attributes. Cattell's crystallized intelligence would be considered as phenotypic intelligence, while fluid intelligence would be genotypic intelligence. In a like manner, "G" intelligence would be more like fluid or genotypic intelligence, while aptitudes would be more like crystallized or phenotypic intelligence.

INTELLIGENCE IN THE BLIND

Blind and visually-impaired children, on average, score the same as sighted children on standardized tests of intelligence. This strongly supports the notion that vision loss does not impair fluid or genotypic intelligence. In other words, visually handicapped children have the same intellective processes available to them to use in coping with their particular environments.

Will Beth Stephens and Kathy Simpkins conducted research on the cognitive development of blind children compared to sighted children as measured by various types of Piagetian tests. They found that, on average, blind children scored from four to eight years behind sighted children on all but one of these tests even though they had the same measured intelligence based on I.Q. tests. The differences on the Piagetian tasks increased with age.

In later research, these same two researchers demonstrated that most of these deficits could be successfully remediated using particular and specialized rehabilitative and educational interventions (They were unable to remediate deficits in spatial awareness).

It is interesting to speculate that the differences in the performance on the Piagetian tasks represent phenotypic or aptitude differences but not genotypic differences. It is certainly possible, however, that just the opposite is true. This would be a useful area for further research.

It should be clear that vision loss is not the only factor which can affect cognitive development. Specifically, much has been written on the relative intelligence of racial and ethnic minorities and females and males. Most studies (though not all) have found that, on average, individuals in these groups have I.Q.s that are about the same. When individual aptitude tests are used to measure specific abilities, however, differences are observed. Might it be possible that "G" intelligence is the same in these groups and accounts for the similarities while aptitude or crystallized intelligence accounts for the differences?

Many studies of twins, both identical and fraternal, reared together and reared apart, as well as studies of children with different hereditary relationships, tend to show a strong relationship between measured intelligence and level of relatedness. Only a small fraction (between 10% and 15%) of the variance is unexplained on the basis of genetic factors. The authors are not aware of any studies which have compared levels of relatedness and scores on aptitude tests. If such studies were conducted, they might show that specific differences in the environments would explain more differences than when "average" or typical I.Q. scores are used.

DISCUSSION

As noted above, definitive answers to questions concerning the relative contributions to development of heredity and environment are not possible at this time. As a result, you may leave this chapter with more questions than you had when you started it. This is not something to be too concerned about if you have come away with an increased awareness of the complexity of the issues. You certainly need to know your own biases as you work in your profession, and you should be alert for new information bearing on this issue throughout your career.

SUGGESTED READINGS

1. Hebb, D.O., & Thompson, W.R. (1954). The social significance of animal studies. G. Lindsay & E. Arouson (Eds.), *The handbook of social psychology*, vol. 2 (2d ed.). Boston: Addison-Wesley, pp. 729-774.
2. Piaget, J. (1952). *The origins of intelligence in children.* New York: International Universities Press.
3. Stephens, B., & Simpkins, K. (1974). The reasoning, moral judgment, and moral conduct of the congenitally blind: Final Project Report, H23-3197. Washington, DC: Office of Education, Bureau of Education for the Handicapped.

Chapter 5

SCIENCE AND THE VISUALLY IMPAIRED

INTRODUCTION

In this chapter, we will seek to demonstrate relationships between commonly held scientific assumptions and various theories and approaches used in work with the blind and visually limited. The discussion will include how these assumptions relate to problems associated with visual handicaps. The focus of this chapter is the usefulness of scientific thinking in trying to develop a foundation for a "psychology of blindness." or "sociology of blindness."

The application of the scientific methods for understanding the world in which we live is undisputed, especially for understanding the physical world. However, scientific methodology has been far less successful in providing useful knowledge in human affairs. The failure to achieve the same success in social areas as in the physical domain probably stems from some of the basic, underlying, philosophical assumptions used by scientists. If these assumptions were broadened and clarified, it might be possible to make greater contributions to comprehending human beings and the social and psychological world in which they exist and improve our ability to understand the problems related to vision loss.

Among many, there are five assumptions made by scientists. Often these assumptions are used implicitly and perhaps even unconsciously. Each assumption obviously cannot be discussed in detail to discover all of their implications, but this listing will provide the basis for the discussion which is included here. Here are the assumptions with a brief discussion of each.

1. It is assumed that the world and all in it are capable of being understood. This assumption implies that we can observe all of reality and that the various parts of that reality are harmonious and fit into a general framework of facts. We may not know all of the methods which will yield understanding, we are told, but if we persist, understanding will come as it has in the physical world.

An opposing assumption could be that the world is not understandable, a position known as "skepticism." Those who favor this position point out that we can observe only a tiny part of the universe, both in the microcosm and the macrocosm at any one time. No one can observe all of the universe simultaneously, and even if one could observe everything happening at any point in time, he/she could not describe all the events taking place completely. In addition, one must assume that all past and future events are guided by the same regularities as those events occurring at our point in time. This opposing assumption is very pessimistic, while assumption A is optimistic.

2. A second assumption holds that at the very foundation of all reality is a single, fundamental principle or law which explains and guides all existence. This assumption guides the thoughts and studies of those who seek to form a "Grand Unifying Theory" (GUT). This implies the laws we observe are only partially valid, but to the extent they are useful, they will conform to the more fundamental presumed law. It is further assumed that, as we continue to "chip" away at this huge universe and its fundamental operations we will eventually discover the essentially simple, foundational truths.

3. A third assumption is that the world is governed by at least a few general principles or laws which, if understood, would make the world understandable and predictable. As with assumption A some scientists and philosophers of science argue that "natural laws" do not actually exist, but that they are creations of man to simplify his world; but the world is constantly in a state of change which is never exactly repeated. These individuals point to several problems that complicate our efforts to discover these basic truths. Some of these problems are:

   (a) There is such a short time during our lives to work at discovering truth. The Universe is so old—at least 15 billion years—

and our lives so short that we cannot see patterns or continuities.

(b) The Universe is so vast, and we are so tied to our tiny planet, that we can observe only superficially what it is like. This is the macrocosm. In the opposite direction—the microcosm—we can observe only relatively large objects. In the atomic and subatomic world there is another vast world which defies our unaided observations.

(c) The Universe at the surface is so complex and variable—no two things are exactly the same—that seeing underlying patterns and relationships is extremely difficult. This difficulty may be summed up by a paraphrase of Einstein's famous observation that God is not malicious, but He is subtle.

(d) Results obtained by one discipline such as astronomy, physics, or sociology, for example, are very difficult to explain in ways that other disciplines can understand and appreciate. Instead of contributing to a common understanding of the fundamental reality, each discipline works in its own narrow domain and in different directions.

4. Still another assumption is that matter and energy represent the whole of reality and that there is no need to consider other, nonobservable aspects of life which have been used in the past such as the concepts of mind, thought, spirit, etc. In other words, by assuming a strictly materialistic universe, many other aspects of potential reality have been placed off limits for our investigations.

5. A more restrictive assumption is that all phenomena can be reduced to physical processes such as chemistry or physics. This assumption of "materialistic reductionism" has a seemingly positive objective, i.e., simplifying our world. However, it makes understanding human behavior very difficult, if not impossible, and, it is not a reasonable assumption since some aspects of the universe have no material evidence.

None of these assumptions is provable. And, some of them have unnecessarily limited investigations of the behavior of human beings. They have been very useful, as noted above, in dealing with the physical universe, but they have been less useful in such fields as education and psychology. We will feel free to make other assumptions if we find such assumptions useful in understanding that part of the universe in which we are most interested.

OBJECTIVES

At the completion of this chapter readers will be able to

1. Identify assumptions which guide scientific research. Readers will realize that research foci do not choose themselves and that assumptions direct and limit the questions we seek answers for.
2. Modify basic research assumptions in order to broaden them to facilitate finding answers to questions about the effects of vision loss on learning, motivation, and other psychological processes.
3. Define the terms "ideographic," "nomothetic," "convergent thinking," and "divergent thinking" and relate them to rehabilitative and educational organizations and methods.
4. Recognize and describe reasons for continued research to encourage discovery of new facts related to the education and rehabilitation of those with vision loss.

THE VIENNA CIRCLE

Just before World War I, a group of educational philosophers (The Vienna Circle) met together on a regular basis in Vienna, Austria to establish a standard against which a statement could be judged for its meaning. They arrived at what was referred to as "The Empirical Standard of Meaning." A statement was meaningful only if it could be verified through direct observation or if it was logically self-evident. The first criteria limits meaningfulness to statements which describe sensory information alone. This is referred to as "radical empiricism" or "logical positivism." The second part refers to a statement based on logical grounds such as 2 x 2 = 4. This kind of statement is essentially circular or tautological reasoning because nothing other than the logical rule is added.

This group of proponents of "radical empiricism" and of "logical positivism" broke up when its members took teaching positions at some of the most prestigious universities in Europe and in America. Several generations of teacher-educators learned at their feet. Their belief that only observable phenomenon or self-evident logic is meaningful led to the general adoption and use of behavioral principles and instructional strategies in our schools.

It is interesting to note that the statement of the "Vienna Circle's" principles is, itself, nonmeaningful according to their criteria being neither self-evident or directly observable. Further, few statements used in religion, education, sociology, ethics, etc. would have any meaning if this standard were used.

The principles developed and disseminated by this group were highly influential in the revolution which took place in education and psychology which followed. This revolution was part of a much broader change which took place in almost all other facets of science, law, medicine, philosophy, and ethics during the nineteenth century and the first part of the twentieth century. The revolution involved a revolt against the influence of religious thought on our entire society. Laws passed by legislative bodies and which were based to a great extent on the Ten Commandments and other Judeo-Christian principles were reinterpreted to reduce or eliminate these influences. The various sciences sought "natural" explanations for the world and the universe. Darwin's theory of organic evolution, it was assumed, eliminated the need for an external, super-human involvement in the development or creation of life in its myriad forms. Ethics and concepts of morality were explained in terms of pragmatic, secular concepts which eschewed theistic surveillance. The scientific investigations of men such as Newton and Descartes were stripped of references to the religious views of the investigators.

While this secularization of intellectual thought was taking place, the public at large continued to accept the older biblical/creationist world view. While it is true that many of the great thinkers of this era were personally involved in religious practices and adhered to religious and ethical principles, their professional endeavors were stripped of the religious influences. This was done, ostensibly to be more objective and less irrational than thinkers from the past.

The change in the Zeitgeist was gradual and subtle, but it led to the development of theories which have influenced views of the general public as well as those who occupy intellectual circles. Freud popularized the notion that children's character and intellectual development were brought about by interactions between parents and their children, especially where "pathology" was concerned. He replaced the idea of a soul which was capable of making and acting upon conscious choices with a naturalistic interaction of biological processes and environmental influences. Since these biological and social interactions were beyond the control—or even the influence—of the individual, a person is not responsible for his/her actions.

RADICAL EMPIRICISM

Radical empiricism is closely related to philosophical realism and has influenced the development of many rehabilitative and educational innovations. As noted in other chapters, this approach dominates modern rehabilitative and educational practice, even though its tenets have largely lost favor in the physical and biological sciences. In recent years, many researchers have expanded their thinking to include the possibility of factors which cannot account for observed phenomena such as conscience, spirit, and a creative power. These modern intellectuals have found that radical empiricism is too limiting of research in areas of human psychology, education, and behavior.

Marshall McLuen quoted a poem by an unknown author which seems to summarize the nature of many current assumption:

In Modern Thought, if not in fact,
Nothing is that does not act.
So THAT is reckoned wisdom which
Describes the scratch, but not the itch.

Those concepts which most clearly distinguish human being from other creatures such as "mind," "thought," "perception," "honesty," "intelligence," "consciousness," "purpose," "will," "morals," etc. are not directly observable, and, therefore, according to this assumption, are not within the scope of science.

Although these aspects of psychology are not, in fact, directly observable, they can be inferred from experiments which produce observable behaviors. For example, Meltzoff has studied the behaviors of 18-month-old infants who observe the actions of adults, and then when they are placed in the position of the adult, the child imitates the actions of the adult in trying to accomplish a task or reach a goal. When a mechanical robot demonstrated the task, however, the child does not typically attempt to achieve the goal. In other words, the child infers the intent of the adult and attempts to achieve the same purpose. Nothing, even the most accurate observations by sophisticated instruments, can begin to explain why two individuals having the same experience react in different ways.

INFERRED REALITY

Consider the following information as a contrast to the above. If you observe a chemical process in action, or you observe the weather, do your observations in any way alter the chemical process or the weather? Anyone watching these phenomena does not alter them. In other words, aspects of the physical world are not "aware" that they are being watched.

In contrast, suppose a person goes into a fifth-grade class to observe from the back of the room, will the observations influence the actions of the students? Even though changes in behavior can be observed due to the presence of a new person, can you, from a logical-positivistic standpoint, describe the mechanisms of influence? Does this kind of observation require any "intervening variable" or inferred factors in order to account for these differences? What if the children were all totally blind and you did not make any sounds as you entered the classroom? Would the variation from nonobserved behaviors be accounted for by the sight stimuli themselves? It would seem that something more than the stimuli per se are necessary to explain what was happening.

Even though this is a simple example, it has profound implications for scientific procedures. It is virtually impossible, on the basis of direct observations, to reduce the observed differences to purely mechanical or physical processes. The difference in the reactions of clients and chemical elements marks the differences between psychological factors and physical factors alone. To put it a different way, something more is involved than can be directly observed, e.g., the ability of human beings to understand and to make decisions and choices based on that understanding. These are inferred rather than being directly observed. Even in the physical sciences, however, most concepts are not directly observed, but are also inferred. For example, no one has directly observed such entities as quarks, nuons, gravity, force fields, etc. We infer their existence on the basis of the effects they have on other things which we can observe.

If we are to make progress in understanding human psychological and sociological functioning, we must alter the assumptions we use in research in order to study variables which must be inferred, and a strictly behavioral science of education is a gross oversimplification of this reality.

In the earlier history of psychology, a concept was used to describe and explain some aspects of actions known as "Conation." This term covered such things as intentions, purposes, or will. In philosophical parlance, the term "teleology," which implies the idea that the intentions of people is a simpler and more parsimonious explanation than trying to establish an inferred cause-and-effect chain of events.

BALANCING IDEOGRAPHIC AND NOMOTHETIC MODELS

We observe a world which is infinitely complex, in which no two objects, persons, or events are exactly alike. The idea that everything is, in fact, unique is referred to as the "ideographic model." In contrast, the idea that there are simple, powerful, underlying processes at work is referred to as the "nomothetic model." In other words, the nomothetic approach seeks to reduce the complexity of the world by finding fundamental natural laws.

A process which is used in seeking a unique or specific solution to a problem is "convergent thinking." This process seeks to reduce the unknown elements of a problem to something which is known. The solution is seemingly the only one logic will allow us. In contrast, the problem-solving approach known as "divergent thinking" is used in brain-storming solutions to problems where as many potential, tentative solutions are generated as possible without looking for a single, unique solution.

These two processes are not antagonistic, but complementary, as are the ideographic and nomothetic models. The divergent and ideographic approaches provide us with freedom to explore and to be creative, while the convergent and nomothetic approaches simplify and clarify an otherwise chaotic world often to the exclusion of providing solutions to unique situations. The real issue is one of balance in which we use these processes appropriately without going to the extremes of anarchy or totalitarianism.

In seeking solutions to problems arising in attempting to educate individual children, teachers tend to use divergent and ideographic approaches. Administrators, on the other hand, tend to think of children and teachers in broad, homogeneous groups and seek nomothetic solutions. Their goals relate to establishing smooth-running systems in which fairness and stability are emphasized. Both approaches are very useful unless one of them gets out of balance. If, for example, the teacher is so creative that her class becomes disruptive, or the principal is so concerned about fairness that he does not allow for meeting individual needs, the system is out of balance.

Scientific research endeavors are of necessity essentially nomothetic and convergent in nature. As noted above, however, if we are to be successful in understanding human beings, and particularly visually-impaired persons, then a good measure of ideographic and divergent thinking needs to be introduced into methods used to identify effective services. This is already happening in other disciplines such as neuropsychology and behavioral genetics, but we need to expand the scope of creativity to work for the blind and visually impaired.

THEORY CHOICES

Every scientific discipline is faced with the necessity of choosing from a large number of theories or paradigms in trying to explain the observed phenomena encountered. Upon what basis are the decisions to be made? As noted earlier, there are no generally accepted criteria or universal truths which can act as a yardstick or standard. One approach which has been widely used in the choice of models or analogs for use in science is the pragmatic notion that a theory is best which generates the most testable hypotheses. The process of testing hypotheses is research. If the research produces results which support or do not support the hypotheses, then new hypotheses can be generated and tested. And, if necessary, the theory can be revised to reflect the data derived from the research.

The models of reality which science has produced are never considered final descriptions of reality. This is because, as mentioned above, we can gather such a small number of observations upon which to build these models. It would be necessary to observe all events occurring in an infinite universe at any point in time, and then be able to do this for all possible points in time if a total picture is to be obtained. Since both of these sets of observations are impossible attainments, we must be content with what we are able to do within our own limitations. And, we should recognize that our theories are very tentative and should not be rigidly considered as a final or unchangeable theory.

"ALL INCLUSIVE-ONE SIZE FITS ALL"

A major problem in the education and/or rehabilitation of the visually impaired is the attempts being made at the systems level to fit all disabled children or adults into a single educational setting: the neighborhood school, or, the provision of rehabilitative services to blind adults in a general agency which serves all disability groupings. Individuals having a disability does not mean that they are all of one kind or that all have the same needs.

A person who is blind has a mobility problem that is far different from a person with an orthopedic disability. Children with visual and children with hearing impairments have a sensory loss but the problems in providing education services are not the same. In point of fact, rehabilitative and educational provisions for these two groups could hardly be more different. Systems that try to design uniform processes to meet the needs of diverse groups are seldom very successful using a nomothetic approach. Within a given disability group, there are such widely differing problems that no single approach would be appropriate for everyone within that group. For example, not all visually impaired individuals should learn Braille, nor be restricted to large type or taped materials for all books they read.

The kinds of information needed, the availability of specific kinds of information, and the feasibility of accessing such information requires that individual preferences and circumstances be considered. Thus, if we were to use a nomothetic approach for problem solutions, we could profoundly limit the rehabilitative and educational opportunities for some persons.

Meeting the needs of all children in a neighborhood school may be equally limiting. For example, if the school has limited access to qualified personnel, lack of adaptive equipment, limited time for instruction in skills not included in the core subjects, and no contact with peers for extracurricular activities, this placement may be far more restrictive than a special program or school that provides access to needed services designed for a particular group of persons with a specific disability.

The need to move closer to a divergent, ideographic approach has been recognized with the passage of federal and state requirements of individual rehabilitation plans (IRPs) for rehabilitation services and individual education plans (IEPs) for special education students. These direct, insofar as possible, that programs meet the unique needs of each child or client. It may be more economical (in the short term) to have all children educated in a neighborhood school, or have a single rehabilitation agency which serves all disability groups, but strong evidence exists which casts doubt over the idea that this simplification—or nomothetic—approach is the most appropriate, efficient, and effective for making it possible for these disabled persons to take their places in the mainstream of American life.

An example from the business world may clarify this idea. Near the beginning of the twentieth century, major corporations in America adopted an organizational structure which emphasized a "top down" management system. Thus, decisions were made by the "board of directors" and the chief executive officer. The products to be produced or the services which were to be marketed were selected from among the options available to the corporation.

These decisions were passed on to "middle management," which was to develop strategies for implementing these decisions. The kinds of materials to be used in a manufacturing process were selected and procured, service patterns were devised, and plans made for selling these services.

The employees who actually produced the products or provided the services were viewed as parts of a larger "machine" in which all components must work together according to the management plan. Workers who produced according to the plan were deemed valuable employees and those who "chose" to do things in their unique ways were considered as poor employees. Innovations were not generally looked upon with favor.

In the past few decades, a shift in perspective has occurred. Japanese corporations were achieving remarkable gains in productivity among their workers that surpassed other industrialized countries. These increases in productivity were associated with a change in management philosophy. The CEO and the Board of Directors still set policy, but the production workers—those at the bottom of the structure—were given freedom to develop and modify production procedures. They were given responsibilities and management was to offer resources as needed and to monitor progress.

American corporations began to adopt this system of decentralization and diversification of responsibilities. Productivity has increased, absenteeism was reduced, and employee morale improved. The best explanation for these improvements is that individual interests and talents were utilized in a more open system. The authoritarian model gave way to a more truly democratic system in which the goals and intentions of individuals was balanced against the interests of the corporation, its leaders, and its shareholders.

At the same time these changes in corporate America were taking place, just the reverse process has been taking place in government-financed, service-delivery systems such as education and rehabilitation agencies. School district consolidations reduced the number of school districts, schools, and programs. Administration increased in size and teachers were given less freedom in choosing curricula and methods for teaching. Rehabilitation agencies were placed under an "umbrella" agency with the expectation that management costs would be reduced. Unfortunately, these expectations have not been realized.

In 1987, about half of the states had specialized agencies serving the visually impaired, while the other half had a general agency which provided services on a noncategorical basis. In that year, 70 percent of the closures among visually impaired persons came from the half of the agencies serving this group exclusively and 30 percent from the general agencies.

Several national studies have been conducted, all of which have demonstrated that there is an "economy of scale," which holds that as a system becomes larger, there is a smaller cost per unit of production. This is not a valid approach when human services are involved. The disabled client or student still requires individualized services, and resources are not usually available to provide time for individualization in an umbrella agency.

In like manner, a visually impaired student in a school setting is in need of the same services whether he/she is in an integrated neighborhood school or in a segregated program. The press for greater economies in the "full-inclusion" model actually reduces the availability of these crucial services. Orientation and mobility, Braille instruction, tutorial services, transition programs, and other vital programs are less likely to be provided in a regular classroom and the promised benefits of greater acceptance by nondisabled fellows (the most often reason given for placement in the mainstream) has not been realized.

DISCUSSION

This chapter has looked at some of the ideas that guide researchers and their basic assumptions. There are those in our society who consider science as the only valid source for truth. But, there are so many limitations to this method–as useful as it is–that it cannot be relied upon to give answers to all of life's questions. Some of the most important aspects of human life are specifically excluded from scientific inquiry such as religion, morality, values, etc. If there is a broad, underlying set of true principles, then there should be no incompatibilities of answers to questions derived from approaches used in conjunction with science such as logic, revelation, ethics, etc. when these are considered together. If there are inconsistencies, then it is because one or the other of the approaches has not attained to a sufficiently valid understanding of reality. And, it may be just as likely that science is in error as that religion is. In other words, we should not let a scientific approach replace our religious and/or intuitive values since each in its own way can give us valid answers to some of life's questions.

What is needed is more rigorous research evaluations of hypotheses derived from our various models which guide our service efforts. We should also remain open-minded to new ideas and not dogmatically insist that "our approach" is the only valid model.

Scientific research has not given us final and complete answers to our problems. But if research bases are expanded, more appropriate assumptions articulated, and rigorous research conducted, we can hopefully make progress in meeting the needs of the individuals with whom we work. As discussed in this chapter, there must be an understanding of the implicit assumptions held by researches. And, a balance between nomothetic and ideographic models of service must be implemented so services meet the needs of individuals who have blindness or low vision.

Chapter 6

MEASUREMENT AND ASSESSMENT

INTRODUCTION

A fundamental process in all scientific endeavors is measurement. Measurements are employed to learn about the attributes or qualities of a particular phenomenon, whether the phenomenon be a chemical, a planet, or a human being. Often scientific progress is tied to the development of a more precise and accurate measuring system.

Measurement has been defined as the process in which we assign numbers to our observations according to rules. The rules are essentially mathematical in nature. Observations are made using a variety of methods, ranging from simple counting of the number of times an event occurs to noting how long it takes chemical elements to combine under highly-controlled circumstances. (Molecules can undergo a chemical change in as short a time as one nanosecond.)

Assessment is a collection of measurement results that describe the state of a phenomenon at a point in time. These data are used to identify problems based on similar data taken at earlier times and circumstances, for example, when a doctor takes a patient's temperature. Many measures of temperature indicate that normal for humans is 98.6 degrees. The doctor then assesses some aspects of the patient's health based on that specific measure.

Assessment may also be used to begin to study phenomena. For example, tests of subject matter may be given and scores noted to find out how much the student knows before a new teaching strategy begins. This initial assessment can later be compared to similar data to determine if change has taken place. In this case, assessment data becomes a baseline on which to evaluate change and for hypothesis about the cause of changes.

For a variety of reasons, measurement in education and psychology have fallen far behind measurement in the natural sciences. One reason is that humans are far more complex than anything the chemist or biologist observes. A second reason is that observers cannot directly observe the brain where learning, seeing, remembering, etc. take place. A third reasons is that it is not known at what level to observe, i.e., at the level of atoms and molecules or at the level of national policy development in government or industry. A fourth, problem in observing is psychologists have not developed indirect measurement techniques which enable the observer to measure accurately and consistently *inferred* processes which underlie most human activities. In other words, psychologists infer that intelligence exists and have developed activities which they believe measure it. However, there is no specific, observable evidence that describes intelligence.

Measurements are used to guide both practical applications of knowledge as well as knowledge-generating processes called research. Some examples of how measurements are used include the following situations. An observer gives an achievement test to see if teachers are being successful in teaching subject matter to students. The teacher measures heights and weights to see if the children in the class are normal or typical of other children of the same age. And, the neurologist or neuropsychologist measures blood flow in the brain while subjects are engaged in a memory task to see which parts of the brain are involved.

In this chapter readers will learn some fundamental principles of measurement, some areas of the education of children with visual handicaps' development, and some general types of measuring instruments or procedures. Readers will develop skill in using these instruments and procedures at a later time. They will also learn, of course, terms which are peculiar to the processes of measurement.

OBJECTIVE

Upon completion of this chapter the reader will be able to:

1. Define such terms as assessment, evaluation, test, standardized test, scales, measures of central tendencies, measures of variability, and measures of relationship.
2. Describe the qualities of a good measuring instrument: validity, reliability, usefulness, cost, etc.
3. Identify and describe the kinds of measurements needed for a variety of educational and rehabilitation activities.
4. Understand the relationship between measurement processes and research.

ASSESSMENT PROCESSES

Assessment is the process by which information about a given person or group of people is collected, organized, and interpreted. Information is gleaned from intelligence tests, achievement tests, observations using questionnaires, rating sheets, inventories, checklists, medical reports, case studies, interviews, physical measurements, etc. All of this information will be of little use unless one can organize it so that he or she can quickly find specific parts of that information. Face sheets, profiles, graphs, case summaries, card files, data bases, spreadsheets, etc. need to be developed on computers for this organizational process. Where norms are available, performances will be compared. Changes from earlier observations will be noted, using profile overlays, score comparisons, etc. In short, information will be interpreted to see trends, patterns, differences, and similarities.

The assessment is perhaps the most important part of planning education programs and rehabilitation services. Accurate and comprehensive assessment, as mentioned earlier, provides a "picture" of the student's or client's current situation and when compared with a goal or expectation identifies the differences which must be addressed between what is and what can or should be. Perhaps the best example of the importance of assessment is the individual education plan (IEP) used in special education programs or the individualize rehabilitation plan (IRP). The education goals, services, and placement should all be derived from the assessment. Records such as profiles, checklists, and test scores are kept and updated each year to show progress. One crucial part of the process is to make sure that all measurement is appropriate for the person's age and takes into account unique characteristic such as learning style and disabilities.

EVALUATION PROCESSES

Evaluation is the process which interprets or makes judgments about individuals based on information collected during the assessment process. This process is not as precise nor as straightforward as assessment, but relies on past experience, professional judgment, reason, and even intuition to form hypotheses. It is an attempt to develop a picture of a person or group which will guide future rehabilitation and educational activities and interventions. It involves making decisions about whether progress is being made toward specific objectives and broad goals. With individuals, evaluations often use past performance and comparisons with peers to project future performance and success.

Admission to university training programs provides an example of the evaluation process. Information is gathered which may included high school grade point average, scholastic aptitude scores, examples of extracurricular participation, and awards. Past performance of the student is compared to the profile of successful students at the university. Then, a judgment is made about the likelihood of this student's success and if it is believed this student will succeed, then admission is granted. As indicated above, this is often a professional judgment. However, such individual traits as determination and work habits may allow a student who does not meet the profile for admission to succeed.

The measures used to evaluate must be valid and reliable in order to successfully evaluate student performance and success. It may be, for example, that high school grades are not a good piece of data to include in the assessment and evaluation. This is especially true for students from different cultures or those with disabilities that limit access to the general education curricula.

VALIDITY AND RELIABILITY

Validity (derived from the Latin word meaning "truth") means the extent to which a measuring procedure accurately depicts what it is designed to measure. A rubber band used as a yardstick would not be valid or accurate. Neither would determining a person's intelligence by looking at his or her facial features or the lines in his or her hands be valid.

There are typically four types of validity considered in establishing a measuring instrument's accuracy: content validity, concurrent validity, predictive validity, and construct validity. The first type, content validity, is determined by comparing the content pattern of items on a test with the subject matter in textbooks, lectures, discussions, etc.

Concurrent validity is determined by correlating scores on one test with scores on a second test designed to measure the same factor. For example, the Wechsler Intelligence Scale for Children (WISC) and the Stanford-Binet Intelligence Scale are both designed to measure the intellectual abilities of school age children. A similar score on each test is an indication of concurrent validity.

Predictive Validity is determined by giving a test, then seeing how it correlates with another kind of performance. Predictive validity answers the question—will success in one activity predict success in another activity. For example, does an admissions test for college indicate/correlate with freshman year grade point average. Another example: does trigonometry predict success as a machinist. Or, does ability to read Braille predict success in employment for a person who is blind?

Construct validity is evaluated in terms of the extent to which a test measures hypothetical ideas or theories, e.g., tests which measure Piaget's proposed stages of development. Piaget observed that children move from preoperational to concrete operational ways of thinking around age seven. He then developed tests of conservation to test his constructed idea of how children think and behave.

Reliability is the consistency with which a test measures whatever it measures. No measuring instrument is perfect, i.e., there is always a certain amount of error in all measures. The more error, the less consistent the measurements will be. The less the error, the higher the reliability of the test.

Several methods are used to determine reliability: split-half, test-retest, item analysis, etc. One split-half method compares or correlates performance of clients or students on the even-numbered items with the odd-numbered items on the same or alternate form of the test. The test-retest approach is a measure of stability of a test over time. The test is given to the same children two weeks apart and then the correlation is computed between the performance on the two administrations. In item analysis, each item on a test is correlated with the total test score. If an item does not have a high correlation with the total score, it will detract from the reliability of the test and will need to be replaced or rewritten.

Cost of a test is an important consideration when deciding which test to use. A medical test may be very accurate, but if it is so expensive that the patient cannot afford it, it will probably not be used. Individually-administered intelligence tests are more valid and reliable than group-administered, paper-pencil tests. Most school districts use the group test as a screening device to identify those for whom an individual test must be administered. This practice is to save the costs associated with administering individual tests to everyone.

Some tests would be good to use but are not generally available. An example is the Haptic Intelligence Scale for the Blind (HIS). But the test is not used enough because of the small numbers of potential clients, so test publishers cannot afford to make it available at a reasonable cost. The Blind Learning Aptitude Test (BLAT) is a good test but is difficult to obtain.

Another consideration in selecting a measuring instrument is the ease of administration. If extensive training and time are involved in test administration for only limited information, then it will not be used most of the time. For example, it may be helpful to use an electroencephalograph study of a child during learning to identify areas of brain dysfunction. However, use of this instrumentation is beyond the skill of most psychologists, even though the information would be very useful.

ALTERNATE TESTS AND PLANNING

From the reading above, it is probably clear that collecting and organizing information for people is not an easy or simple task. This is especially true when developing education and rehabilitation plans for a person who is blind or severely visually impaired. The counselor, educator, case worker, or psychologist will need to start out with simple, immediately-available information for a particular person. Since most individuals with visual handicaps cannot take the group-administered tests used in most testing settings, they will need to administer a test orally to the blind person or have the psychologist do it. This is not the ideal method, but results are usually "in the ball park." Some examples of tests and alternate testing methods are described below.

The Slosson Intelligence Test (SIT) is designed for oral administration by teachers or others who are professionals such as nurses, counselors, or social workers and does not require extensive training. Almost all items would be appropriate for use with a child with visual handicaps, too. The Wide-Range Achievement test is also useful for measuring academic progress. Other more extensive achievement tests have forms which are beneficial in use with children who have a vision loss. A researcher may have to search, but it is possible to get some useful information locally on a particular child. At least some medical information, especially information about vision, should be available.

As the worker with the blind gains in experience and confidence, he or she can get a wider range of information such as family constellations, interests, hobbies, personality traits, etc. As reports prepared by other specialists are read, one will learn how the information can be put together in an organized manner.

A cautionary note should be inserted here. Because of the sensitive nature of much of the information gathered about a child or adult, one must realize that much of this information is privileged, i.e., confidential and should not be shared with others outside the agency or school. It is extremely important that the professional learn to protect such information, both for the student/client as well as for the professional worker. Confidentiality and caution are especially critical since the validity and reliability of most instruments can be poor when used with students or clients with visual impairments.

CORRECT USE OF NUMBERS

As stated above, measurement consists in assigning numbers to observations according to rules. The simplest rules are for lower-order observations, while more complex rules are for higher-order observations. The rules allow the organization of the numbers for analysis. The organization is represented by "scales" or ordering of the information or observations.

The lowest order of scales is the nominal scale in which each observation—whether it is a test score, a student, or a color preference—is given an identification number. No two observations can receive the same designator. (The value of the observation may be the same, but it is still given a separate designation.) An example might be simply assigning each student in a class a number in consecutive order starting with the number one to the number 20 in effect replacing names with numbers.

In the next level—the ordinal scale—the numbered observations are arranged on the basis of an ordering of the magnitude of some characteristic such as a comparison of heights, order of finish in a race, or ranking of preferred foods. Each observation is not only separate, but is ordered in comparison with other observations. The actual magnitude of the score is not considered, only its ranking. For example, the first and second-place runners in a race may be very close while the third-place runner may be well behind, but the order of one, two, and three does not reflect such differences.

The third level is the interval scale. In this scale the separate scores are maintained along with order. But the actual magnitude of each score is added. The Fahrenheit temperature scale is an example. The temperatures are arranged along a fixed comparison line, with magnitude increasing by equal increments as one moves along the line. The intervals are equal, but the line begins at an arbitrary point rather than an absolute or meaningful point. A temperature of 50 degrees is not half the warmth of one hundred degrees so the ratio cannot be determined.

The last scale is the ratio scale. This scale retains the rules for the three other scales but adds a starting point on the comparison line which represents an absolute or meaningful zero point. For example, a weight of 10 ounces is one-third of 30 ounces because the zero point represents the absence of weight. For this reason points along the scale can be compared in terms of the ratio of the values of the observations.

Social security numbers represent a nominal scale; ranking in weight comparisons in a group would be an ordinal scale; scores on an I.Q. test would be an interval scale; and shoe sizes in inches would be a ratio scale. The precision of measurements should be assigned numbers reflecting the kind of data obtained. The investigator must be aware of which scale is appropriate before assigning values such as assigning numbers at an interval-scale level when the observations are of ordinal data.

STATISTICS AND PARAMETRICS

Professionals use the information from the above scales for several purposes but primarily for descriptions and for drawing inferences. The purposes will determine whether he or she merely describes the observations or tries to reason from these observations to conclusions which are not directly observed. The first use is assessment; the second use includes evaluation judgments.

If the numbers are used to describe a sample or a representative subpart of a population, they are referred to as "statistics." If the numbers describe the entire population–every person, object, or event possessing the characteristics used to define the group–they are called "parameters." The three most commonly used statistical and parametric descriptors are measures of central tendency, measures of dispersion or variability, and measures of relationship. The three usual measures of central tendency are the mode, the median, and the mean. The three usual measures of dispersion are the range, the semi-interquartile range, and the standard deviation. The two most common measures of relationship are the Spearman, Rank-Order Correlation Coefficient and the Pearson Product-Moment Correlation Coefficient. It is not the purpose of this text to give instruction in statistical procedures. It is important to know that reporting of information has used the appropriate measures. It is recommended that readers carefully read the definitions of these descriptors. Later they will probably learn how to compute and use them.

It should be noted that the Range and the Mode correspond to nominal-scale data; the Median and the Semi-inter-quartile Range correspond to ordinal-scale data; and the Mean and the Standard Deviation correspond to Interval- and Ratio-scale data. Psychologists use higher-order descriptors for higher-order observations.

There are four more important definitions of measurement terms: parametric inferential statistics, nonparametric inferential statistics, continuous data, and discrete data. If one wants to reason about the parameters of a group (remember the definitions above) from the statistics of a sample, you would use parametric statistical procedures. Examples (with which you do not now need to be concerned) are the t-statistic, analysis of variance and analysis of covariance.

If your sample is not normally distributed (the scores, when tabled, do not form the "normal curve") you will use nonparametric statistical procedures. Examples are chi (pronounced "ky") square and Friedman's analysis of variance.

Discrete data are observations which occur only in whole numbers. Examples would be number of children in a family or state of residence.

Continuous data are observations which may be described as possessing whole numbers and an infinite number of fractional parts of those whole numbers. Examples would be age, weight, and distance.

DISCUSSION

This chapter has presented some basic concepts related to measurement and how measurements are used to assess and plan program for individual education and rehabilitation programs. The definitions and discussion should be helpful whether describing characteristics and needs of a single student or client or planning a research project that will identify needed programmatic changes. Assessment and measurement can also help know when programs are effective.

The concepts described here are applicable to many situations. However, it is often difficult to apply the procedures suggested because (1) the low incidence of people who are blind and the diversity of the population makes it difficult to compare individuals with sighted or blind populations; (2) there are few instruments that are available or appropriate for use with those who have severely limited sight; (3) few professionals have experience with students or adults with vision loss and so cannot interpret findings based on experienced professional judgment. These factors often result in inaccurate assessment and become the cause for poor program planning with poor results for students and clients. Often poor results are evaluated incorrectly and result in "labels" which lead to inappropriate services. Other chapters will discuss other issues related to services. It will become evident how important measurement and assessment are to the education and rehabilitation processes.

SUGGESTED READINGS

1. Scholl, G. T., & Schnur, R. (1976). *Handbook for measurement and evaluation of the visually impaired.* New York: American Foundation for the Blind.
2. Bradley-Johnson, S. (1986). *Psycho-educational assessment of visually impaired and blind students preschool through high school.* Austin, TX: Pro-Ed.

Chapter 7

LEARNING THEORIES

INTRODUCTION

This chapter considers the general frameworks used in developing or choosing a psychological approach for teaching or counseling. There are many theories of psychology as well as theories about many other aspects of education. How should one choose which theory will guide his/her efforts? That is a difficult question to answer because the criteria used are themselves based upon theories.

The decision about the selection of theories is made upon certain philosophical considerations. These considerations, in turn, have occupied philosophers for hundreds and thousands of years, and there is no ultimate basis upon which one can choose among the many approaches available. If one pursues this issue to its logical conclusion, he/she would have to admit that scholars have not clearly defined a universally accepted or apparently final answer.

The authors believe that all of human actions, whether as professionals or, more broadly, as human beings, are based on how one views the world. This includes what is considered reality and how reality has been organized from current experiences compared with the myriad experiences one has had over a lifetime—in short, one's world view. The German word, Veltenschauung, conveys this idea. The "world view" is narrow and provincial, or it can be as broad as life itself. One's own particular world view is unique to each person, though there are many elements or parts of this view which are shared with associates.

OBJECTIVES

At the completion of this chapter the reader should be able to:

1. Cite and describe examples of "idealistic" and "realistic" philosophical approaches to understanding reality.
2. Show a relationship between behavioral and cognitive theories of learning and the philosophical approaches noted above.
3. Recognize the dilemmas which arise from both of these approaches when considering the special circumstances of individuals with visual handicaps.
4. Explain differences in choices of teaching or counseling materials and methods and the acceptance of one or the other of these broad learning theories.

CHOOSING A LEARNING THEORY

Chapter 1 presented an approach which suggested that, because the world is so diverse and complex, people attempt to simplify it through grouping together objects, persons, and events which are distinguishable from one another on the basis of shared or similar attributes into categories. People then respond to individual members of these groups as though they were essentially the same. This approach was not chosen because it is universally accepted, nor because it can be proven to be the best point of view available, but because it is a functional or pragmatic approach which has demonstrated its usefulness.

In this chapter, two broad approaches to understanding learning theories will be presented. There are other approaches which might be used, but there is not enough time nor resources to consider all of these and so, the authors have chosen these two approaches because they represent models which are used by almost all psychologists and educators today, both in their own practices and in textbooks.

These approaches are not part of everyday conversations nor do most people consider them as of vital interest. It would be pleasing to be able to avoid them, but they seem to be essential for understanding various theoretical options in education and rehabilitation. The fact that many teachers and teacher educators, along with others who work with psychological constructs, have not come to grips with these issues may, in part, account for some of the current dilemmas faced in rehabilitation and public education and especially in special education.

IDEALISM

Idealism: Philosophical "Idealism" is based on the belief that people do not have direct access to ultimate reality, i.e., that the world they experience through the senses is not the whole of what the world is like. It holds that reality consists of the ideas which people have formed about the world, which may have been influenced by sense experience, but which in the final analysis are thoughts developed through reason and contained in the structures of the brain given through heredity. In a comparison of views of reality, the readers will find that people have constructed or made their own reality and that each person's construction will be unique but with some strong underlying similarities to the constructions of others.

(NOTE: One alternative approach holds that each individual's conditions are totally unique and are not knowable by others. This is known as "phenomenology." It is not considered as a very useful approach to education, though its assumptions cannot be refuted.)

The ancient Greek philosopher Plato, who lived between 427 B.C. and 347 B.C., is credited with contributing greatly to this approach. Plato held that people have in their minds all knowledge in the form of ideas, and that these ideas are accessible through the process of reason.

Plato gave an analogy which illustrates this view. He said that people are like slaves chained in a cave with their faces to a wall and their backs to the cave opening. Light coming through the cave entrance casts shadows of the truly "real" objects and events of the world which are between their backs and the light. That which they experience with their senses is like the shadows on the cave's wall. Occasionally, a person will free himself from his fetters and will be able to turn around and see the true aspects of reality. Such a person—not surprisingly—according to Plato, is a philosopher.

(NOTE: If Plato had been an engineer, lawyer, school principal, etc., do you think he would have accepted that person's beliefs as his freed viewer?)

Another contributor to Idealistic thought is Emanuel Kant. Like Plato, he questioned whether people can rely on their senses to give knowledge about ultimate reality without the interventions of their minds. They select, order, refine, interpret, evaluate, etc. sensory information and, therefore, are not capable of determining what "raw" information their senses give them. All they are aware of is the final, mind-processed outcomes. In short, he considers what people know as more the product of the mind than of the senses alone.

Kant also provided thinkers with an analogy to assist in understanding his ideas. He says that minds are like a grist mill. The raw grains are brought to the mind by the senses. The grist mill separates the grain into its several components—husks or bran, endosperm, and flour. They cannot observe this separation process. All they can know is the ideas or concepts with which they understand the world. The "original grain" is not directly observable, but only the products which arise from them.

A more modern approach based on the science of physics which supports this viewpoint is both interesting and provocative. There are a number of energy systems which surround people which they have been able to study with sophisticated technologies. One of these energy systems is the "electromagnetic spectrum." The spectrum covers a wide range of divisions that are used for such aspects of life as electricity, radio, television, visible light (including colors), x-rays, gamma rays, and cosmic rays, to mention just a few.

The spectrum is made up of energies, both naturally produced and manmade, characterized by sine waves (see Figure 7.1). These waves differ in the distance between the peaks of two adjacent waves and in terms of the number of waves which pass a given point in space, usually in a period of one second. The term "hertz" means cycles per second.

Electricity as an example has a wave length of approximately 3,000 kilometers, and frequencies as low as one cycle per second to several hundred cycles per second. The AM radio band has frequencies which range from 550 kilocycles (thousands) per second to 1725 CPS (cycles per second or Hertz). Television operates in a band of the Electromagnetic Spectrum, which contains three bands from 54-80 MHz; 147-212 MHz; 480-650 MHz.

There are approximately four quadrillion potential units of the electromagnetic spectrum. A part of this vast spectrum is a small portion

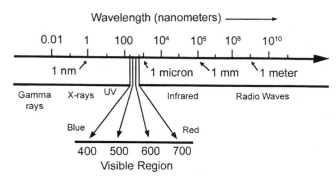

Electronmagnetic Spectrum

Figure 7.1. A complex universe. The light spectrum is only a small part of the vast electromagnetic spectrum found in the universe.

that can be experienced as sight. It is conceivable that there could be sensory and neural systems which would provide the scientist with information from each of these possible parts of the spectrum. They can identify all of the parts of the spectrum with technology, but that is not the same as experiencing these parts as psychological components.

That part of the spectrum which the normal human eye can perceive has wavelengths from 400 to 750 nanometers, with red colors at the longer wavelengths and violet at the shorter wavelengths. Other colors have wavelengths at intermediate points between these two extremes. According to a study conducted by the American Optometric Association, normal eyes can differentiate approximately 7.5 million different colors when they take into account such factors as brightness, saturation, and hue.

Humans also have the ability to perceive objects or events which are highly complex. Even photographs or television pictures convey only a small part of this complexity. The visual system which interacts with the other senses makes possible the interpretation of these recorded stimuli.

A question arises concerning the perception of colors. People who have total "color blindness" can see light, but they do not distinguish colors, but rather see shades of gray with white and black at the extremes. Does color perception reside in the light itself, or is it only a function of the retinas, optic nerves, and the brain? The old question of whether sound occurs in the absence of a hearer when a tree falls in the forest is based on the same issue.

The more important question for educational purposes arises with respect to the parts of the electromagnetic spectrum. If an imaginary line were drawn into space about 5 million kilometers (or 3 million miles) long to represent the Electromagnetic Spectrum, the part which would represent visible light would be one-half inch on that line. Humans do not have sensory systems to perceive the rest of the spectrum, and they know of the other parts of the spectrum through technology. This means that they have no physical-psychological mechanisms for receiving information from this vast array of energy that exists.

In the mind (imagination) they can project a vector (line) into space to infinity. There would be an infinite number of events which occur along this vector. They cannot observe all of these events. And, they could draw an infinite number of vectors into space, each with an infinite number of events occurring along its length.

It has been argued that they have no way of knowing about these events except to assume that they are of the same character as those events they observe in this tiny corner of the universe. When a time-frame is superimposed upon these events, they are forced to attempt to describe them in terms of these minuscule time and space perspectives. This state of affairs poses a real dilemma: they cannot be certain that any knowledge they have developed on earth is valid, and they are without any means of ascertaining its validity or truthfulness. Explorations into the Universe might contradict local truths.

There are many other contributors to this school of thought that cannot be dealt with here. The approach, however, is evident today in "Cognitive Field" theories in psychology (as well as in many other disciplines). Some of the best known theories based on the Idealist notions are those of Jerome Bruner, David Ausebel, Jean Piaget, and Morris L. Bigge.

REALISM

Realism: Philosophical "Realism" is generally credited to another ancient Greek philosopher, Aristotle, who was a student of Plato and the mentor of Alexander the Great. Unlike Plato, Aristotle held that most knowledge of reality comes from the senses. Differences among people result from failure to observe closely enough or extensively enough. Knowledge increases as the direct increase in the accuracy and extent of observations shared between and among humans. The ultimate test of reality is sensory information.

Another contributor to the Realist position was John Locke. He argued that at birth the mind is completely blank, like a clean chalkboard. As the senses bring information into the mind, "marks" are made on the "chalkboards" and as more and more marks are made, the picture of reality becomes clearer and clearer. According to this point of view, people are passive recipients of the environment in which they find themselves. They cannot go beyond the information written upon their minds by the senses.

The modern psychological theories, which are based on Realism's conception of the world, include the broad field of "Behaviorism." Specific theories in this area are those of Ivan Pavlov, Clark Hull, John B. Watson and B. F. Skinner. These theories have dominated educational thought for the past half century, but cognitive field theories have become increasingly popular over the past decade as behavioral theories have waned.

One major appeal of the Realistic approach is its affinity to modern science and the desire to make education more like the physical and biological sciences. Although they use research methodologies in education, they have not been nearly so productive of useful knowledge as they have in other fields. The enigmas of human psychology have not yielded to scientific inquiry, based solely on observable phenomena. And, as a result, they have many "facts," but nothing which resembles the "laws" which other disciplines have developed. The subject matter of human behavior with which they deal is infinitely more complex than the physical world, and science has found no way to apply its observational methods to the study of some of man's most characteristic concerns such as morality, character, values, religion, free will, etc. While they will continue to use scientific approaches, they should be exploring additional construct systems which, more and more, are based on the broader Idealistic paradigm.

APPLICATION OF LEARNING THEORIES

Since the 1970s, most texts have pointed out the similarities and differences between these two broad approaches, though authors may slant their presentations toward one approach or the other. When students begin a course of study that includes a relatively new textbook in educational psychology, he/she should read the introductory chapters and the chapters dealing with learning theories.

It is important for teachers and other professionals who plan for training of children and adults to not only understand learning theories but to deliberately choose and believe in a personal philosophy of education that is consistent with their knowledge. Consistency and commitment are essential ingredients in rehabilitation and education processes. Using methods that have their basis in Realism when values and activities are based on concepts from Idealism will likely be very frustrating to both the teacher and the student. This is because expectation for classroom management, student discipline, choice of materials, use of field trips, etc. are guided by the instructors's philosophy. Any person seeking employment in human services, including education and rehabilitation, should attempt to see if their philosophy and the philosophy of the employing organization are a close match.

An example may help understand the need for a personal philosophy. Suppose that a blind person begins a course under the direction of a teacher and organization of the Realism persuasion. Success would likely be based on completion of a rather rigid set of behavior objectives. There would be specific methods for teaching the course. Recitation of information of thoughts presented by the instructor would predominate. Teachers would be the "dispensers" of knowledge. Students would have little choice in what, how, and when they were taught. Rigid rules of the organization would be a hallmark of the program.

A program based on Idealism would differ in many respects. Students would be regarded as the learners with teachers as facilitators. Organization rules and patterns would seem less obvious to allow for different styles of learning. Recitation would consist of discussion of concepts related to achievement of individual goals. Activities would expect students to "discover" how to accomplish tasks and gain new knowledge.

The point to be gained is not to indicate that one philosophy is to be used to the exclusion of all others. Rather, each instructor needs to understand the benefits of each one used and also be aware of the limitations. To illustrate, there are perhaps very specific methods for teaching touch typing to a blind or visually impaired person. This course may well benefit from a very rigid method, and specific behavioral objectives. However, the same person may need a significant amount of discussion to understand concepts related to adjusting to being blind. In other words, there are some subjects that lend themselves to each of the general learning theories. However, caution should be exercised since reliance on "discovery" in subjects such as orientation and mobility will be dangerous. And, dogmatic answers to developing self-esteem thwart true feelings and creativity.

Probably no individual follows a purely Realist or Idealist position, but everyone is more eclectic. However, they must be conscious of their philosophical position. To emphasize the point, professionals must understand the basis of learning theories they are taught, examine their personal philosophy, and try to be consistent in their applications to specific course content.

EXAMINING ONE'S PERSONAL PHILOSOPHY OF LEARNING

Professionals who work with children and adults who are blind or visually impaired, like all other people, already have personal philosophies. And, it is just as important, or maybe more so, that they identify whether Realism or Idealism is their basis for developing and using particular methods and materials with those who do not see normally. It may even be that after thorough consideration an individual may find that his or her beliefs do not lend themselves to work with the blind.

As mentioned in an earlier chapter, absence of sight forces the person who is blind to form concepts based on more inductive thinking than those with normal sight. The necessity of inductive thinking would seem to be an example of Plato's analogy of only seeing shadows on the cave wall. The blind person only encounters what he or she can touch, smell, taste, hear, and to what degree the distance sight is limited. The sensory limitations limit the world. However, through inductive reasoning accurate concepts can be formed. Each new sensory experience or discussion based on experience leads to the opportunity for new, better and more accurate concepts.

Therefore, successful teaching of a blind person is of necessity a mixture of Realist and Idealist strategies. In the early stages of learning, such as preschool and early elementary grades, it is important to provide as much real experience as possible. Later, initial concepts can be altered by symbolic methods to refine concepts or develop new ones. As mentioned above no single individual will or should use one type of instruction or learning theory to the exclusion of all else. However, different ages and stages of blind learners require specific techniques drawn from Realism and Idealism philosophies and learning theories based on these root beliefs at different times and for different subject matter.

Those who seek education and rehabilitation services should talk to one or more teachers in his/her local schools or agencies that provide training programs for the blind and find what theoretical approach they tend to agree with. Ask specifically what the program's philosophy of service is. If it is not possible to understand the underlying basis for activities and objectives, ask how choices are made as to what is to be taught, to whom it is to be taught, i.e., to everyone, to first graders, etc.—and what methods are to be used. If a "one size fits all" is used for all ages and/or degrees of vision loss, appropriateness of the program should be questioned.

DISCUSSION

If the reader has an interest in further study of the philosophical background of these approaches, he/she should try to find books such as John D. Cannon's *World Within the World,* which delves into the issue from the broad scientific viewpoint or Morris L. Bigge's *Learning Theories for Teachers* which explores the more limited implications for teachers. These references will be helpful in gaining understanding and perhaps in discovering a personal philosophy of education and rehabilitation.

There are entire textbooks and courses that deal with the issues briefly presented here. The discussion in this chapter has focused only on the two most common philosophical orientations. It is anticipated that the reader will consider this chapter as only a beginning of the reader's study of learning theories and their relevance for education (especially education of children and adults with visual handicaps), rehabilitation, life, and its survival.

SUGGESTED READINGS

1. Aristotle. (1997). *Politics.* translated by Peter L. Phillips Simpson. University of North Carlina Press.
2. Plato. (1985). *The Republic.* New York: W. W. Norton.

Chapter 8

THE SENSES AND PERCEPTION

INTRODUCTION

Human beings are "marvelously made." Their bodies and minds make it possible for them to live and function in an extremely complex world, to both learn about this world and to emotionally appreciate it. All of this is possible because of their senses and their brains.

In this chapter, readers will obtain an overview of the senses, particularly the visual system. Readers will see how the various sensory systems interact and overlap to provide an amazing quantity of information which people must learn to understand and interpret. Readers will also be introduced to what it means to a person when one or more of the sensory systems are lost or damaged, and how other sensory systems and the brain can substitute for information thus lost.

The process by which sensory information is organized, interpreted, and used is perception. Readers will be provided an overview of this process, especially as the process is affected by vision loss.

The major goal of this chapter is to provide an overview of how vision loss impacts perception, to assist the student in understanding the kinds of information provided by vision, and to provide the student with preliminary information concerning substitute sources of information through other sensory modalities. Readers will then look more closely at the visual system and learn to identify the parts of this system. This will be only an overview, however. The physiology or functioning of the visual system will be left for another course, but this overview in the present chapter will enable you to understand materials which will be presented in this and other chapters.

OBJECTIVES

At the completion of this chapter readers will be able to:

1. Identify and name the principle parts of the eye.
2. Describe the kinds of information received through the eye.
3. Recognize how different eye defects restrict the amount of information available to a person with visual impairments.
4. Identify and describe substitute sources of information through other modalities which permit near-normal functioning.
5. Understand the nature and benefits of redundancy in sensory and perceptual systems.
6. Recognize that the brain is involved in the organization and interpretation of sensory information received from the senses.

THE NERVOUS SYSTEM

The parts of the body involved in receiving, interpreting, storing, and using information from the environments are the sensory systems and the brain. Typically these are taken for granted unless a person finds him/herself in a situation where one or more of the senses cannot function properly as in a dark and noisy room. People habitually use information coming to their brains without much thought of how they acquired these habits. One burns a fingertip and is not able to feel the texture of the surface of a table, or one goes to the eye doctor for an examination and cannot see detailed material such as print for several hours while the drugs used to dilate or enlarge the pupil wear off. These experiences help one appreciate how much they depend on their senses. They still do not understand or remember the long time it took themselves, as infants and children, to learn how to use their eyes, hands, tongue and nose. They also do not think about the processes in learning about the things around and within them.

The receptors by which the senses provide information from the environments–the social and physical world outside our bodies and our inner-body workings–are essential for life and learning. They have been referred to (and rightfully so) as "Gateways to the Mind." It is common knowledge that humans have five senses–vision, hearing, touch, taste, and smell—but it is not so well known that they have many other senses including the kinesthetic, balance, hunger, thirst, etc. senses.

Energy sources such as light or sound waves, both inside and outside the body, activate receptor cells, as in the retina of the eye, the skin, on the tongue, etc., which then send a signal over the nerve's synapses and fibers to the brain. The signal moves along the nerve fiber at different rates, depending on the size of the fiber. Larger fibers connect the brain with body extremities which carry the signals more rapidly than the thin fibers which connect the face or other senses closer to the brain. The speed of the signal is calibrated in such a way that a signal from the foot and from the ear which arises from the same external energy source arrive at the brain at the same time. If this were not so, the brain would not be able to know that the signal from the toe and the sound from the ear arose from the same event.

The signal is referred to as a stimulus and the body has about one million of these signals or stimuli arriving in the brain every second. The signals are sorted and sent to specific locations in the brain such as the center for seeing or the center for feeling. These centers are called "sensory projection areas."

The signals transmitted along each nerve fiber are essentially the same, i.e., signals traveling along the optic nerves are the same as those traveling along the auditory nerves. Humans experience these signals as sights and sounds because of the projection areas (parts of the brain associated with specific sensory processes) rather than because the "message" on each nerve is different. Each signal is an "on-off" signal. The number of signals and the duration of the signals is a function of the stimuli which trigger them. Humans experience the sounds of music because sound waves trigger signals in tiny hair-like nerve endings in the inner ear. The different pitches result from the different nerve endings being activated. The loudness of the sound results from the number of nerve endings activated. But the brain interprets the sounds as melodies or noise.

The signals themselves are electrochemical in nature. The energy which travels along the nerve fiber is generated within the nerve fiber itself. After this self-generated energy is used for a single signal, the nerve fiber must be "recharged" before it can fire again. It is the sequential discharging and charging of this energy which is, in fact, the signal. It is as though you flipped an electric switch. A surge of power moves along the line. You must wait a period of time for another surge of power to be generated before you can flip the switch again for the next signal.

Nerve fibers can discharge and recharge approximately 100 times per second, or one hundred cycles per second or Hertz. As a matter of fact, household electricity—alternating current or A.C. current—operates in the same way at 60 Hertz or 60 cycles per second of on-off surges.

THE VISUAL SENSE

The largest and most information-rich sensory system is vision. There are about 100 million receptors in each retina. These receptors are activated by different wave lengths of light which are typically experienced as different colors. Longer waves are experienced as red; shorter as blue, with all the other colors in between from intermediate frequencies. The intensities or brightness of light results from the number of receptor cells active at any moment.

People do not "see" with their eyes, but rather with the projection areas located in the back part of the brain named occipital lobes and on the sides of the brain, temporal lobes. These projection areas receive the signals and interpret them in terms of pictures. These pictures, in turn, consist of awareness of size, shape, color, lightness, darkness, texture, orientation, etc. and combinations of these. Each characteristic has its own set of receptors in the retina and projection areas in the brain.

Some of the same processes can also be observed by signals traveling over other sensory systems such as touch. The receptors which are stimulated by touch send signals to projection areas of the brain which use texture, temperature, pressure, size, etc. to form a sensation and interpret it.

Seldom does one experience information coming into the brain from a single sensory modality alone. Rather, they get information from several senses simultaneously. For example, they *see* an automobile going by at the same time they *hear* its motor and maybe *feel* vibrations from the ground and *smell* odors from the exhaust pipe. They draw from their memories of similar objects and events which make it possible for the brain to comprehend what the object is and what it is doing.

The reception of signals, their transmission over nerve fibers, and their activation of cells in the projection areas of the brain is referred to as "sensation." The comparison of signals or messages from several sense modalities, retrieval of information from memory and the interpretation of this information are referred to as "perception." Humans usually have the ability to describe each part of an experience in terms of the visual or auditory or tactual information, but more typically, the various sensations are combined into a perception allowing the person to experience the object or event as a whole.

As indicated earlier the human brain is processing an enormous number of signals every second. By multiplying 100 hertz times hundreds of thousands of nerves sending signals to the brain one can gain at least some idea of the quantity of "binary switches" that must be activated, coordinated, "cognized," and interpreted within the brain.

Every sense is important whether it provides information about the outside world (the five sense we most generally think of) or the other senses that maintain operations of the body such as heart rate, breathing, blood sugar levels, hormone level, etc. Vision and the other perceptions are more than a simple transmission of signals that trigger direct responses to specific organs or muscles. Hearing, touch, smell, and taste along with information from the eye is combined with other sensations and categorized or compared with previous memories to form concepts. However, because the retina of the eye transmits such a high number of signals to so many different projection centers in the brain, vision appears to have a dominant role in coordinating messages from many other outside receptors.

THE EYE

The front end organ of seeing is the eye. It receives light from the environment, focuses the light on the retina and generates the sensory signals in the cells of the retina. The eye also can be turned to locate a light source quickly and easily, without moving the head. The parts of the eye work together to bring about the visual sensation process. The parts of the eye which you should know are identified in Figure 8.1.

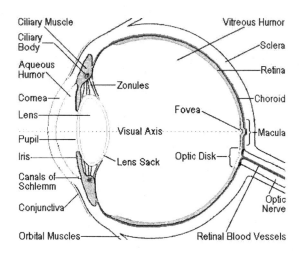

Figure 8.1. The human eye. The parts of the eye work together to convert light waves that create the visual sensation process.

Readers should be able to identify each of these on an unlabeled diagram of the eye, such as the one in your text. Readers should also be able to describe the role played by each in the transformation of light coming from the outside into the projection center for vision—information sent as signals over the optic nerve. It is also important to know what would happen to the light if various parts of the eye are destroyed or defective. For example, if the cornea and/or lens are opaque, light cannot pass through them. If these same two parts are distorted, the light will also be distorted—a condition known as "astigmatism." If the retina is nonfunctional, the light focused on it will not be able to generate nerve-fiber signals for transmission to the visual projection area, etc.

ADAPTATIONS FOR MISSING SENSES

When any sense is missing the organism will not function as well as the development of a normal genetic blueprint of the species would permit. The cause of a physical loss may be either a prenatal mutation, congenital malformation, or trauma that may occur any time during the life of the individual. The time and cause determine to some extent the degree of disability which will result from the impairment.

However, the results will depend on individual situations. For example, animals born with missing limbs often survive by strengthening other body parts in order to forage and do things common to their species. Even when an animal is seriously injured and limbs are amputated, they learn alternative ways to go about life. It is amazing how strongly the instincts and drives push toward "normal" function and activity in the animal kingdoms.

Like all members of the animal kingdom, humans have a genetically determined blueprint for sensory input and many automatic systems and reflexive responses. Fortunately, what distinguishes humans from other animals is the ability to think of responses to impairments rather than merely act by instinct or reflex which gives a wider range of environments where we can be successful. Even going beyond the individual's ability to overcome the effects of disability society has developed education and rehabilitation systems to aid in the normalizing processes.

Education and rehabilitation for the blind and severely visually impaired provide a model for exploring the effects on individuals when a single sensory system is absent or damaged. The visual sense has probably been studied more than any other because of the attitudes toward blindness and the fears associated with becoming blind. Hopefully what is presented next can be helpful in understanding sensory loss in general and will also be helpful to professionals who work with individuals who are blind or have low vision.

The impact of vison loss varies because of many factors such as the age of onset (congenital or adventitious). For example, how to teach and how a child learns who has never had sight is quite different from an adult who has had a lifetime of experiences and visual memories. In fact, studies have shown that there are differences in learning for those who lose their vision before age two, those with sight until five, and\ teens and adults who lose their sight later in life.

There is no doubt that the loss of sight will have an impact and foil natural functioning for an individual. The question for professionals who work with the blind is "Can the effects of vision loss be totally overcome and if so, how?" As mentioned in other chapters, the attitude of the professional will determine what and how services will be provided. Therefore, a theoretical model is presented here that may provide an answer and justify the efforts and costs of educators and rehabilitation workers to those who make and enforce policies and

The Effects of Sensory Loss

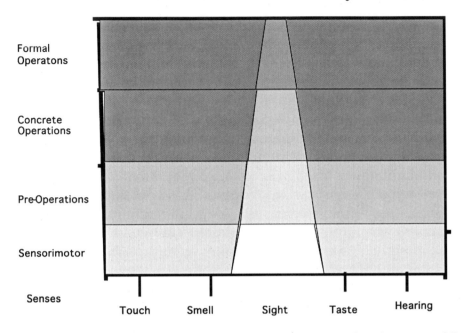

Figure 8.2. Missing sense of sight. Lack of eyesight (represented in the center of Figure 8.2) creates changes in cognitive development that can largely be overcome through later education and rehabilitation training.

allocate funding. The model attempts to illustrate the ability of other senses to take over and change the function of areas of the nervous system and compensate for the lack of specific sensory input and/or projection areas. The words to explain the model are as follows:

When a child is born, it has many systems that contribute to its "normal" development such as sucking reflex, grasping reflex, autonomic nervous system, etc. Each of the systems, along with appropriate food, shelter, and care, is necessary for "normal" development. This is illustrated by the general systems of hearing, touch, taste, etc. shown at the bottom of Figure 8.2. Notice the hole left when the sense of sight is missing. As the child grows, all the remaining systems develop new responses based on genetic unfolding, experience, and training.

As the new responses become available to the child, the brain begins to coordinate the incoming signals and allow them to become coordinated actions that meet needs without the benefit of the input from the visual systems. Notice the beginning of an overlapping of the responses.

At this time, other senses may utilize portions of the brain intended for use as visual projection areas. Later, as the number of interactions between the remaining systems increases, based on experience and training concepts of the world and how it works are formed which allow the individual to accomplish the tasks required by his/her environment and the society in which one lives. Notice the density of the of the interactions increases and the "hole" is less apparent.

At the highest level, the number of connections and concepts is sufficient to make the absence the sense of sight much less significant than at earlier points. Notice that even though the concepts and responses are sufficient they do not have the same density in the area where sight would have provided information and responses.

To give a simple illustration: An adult who has never had even light perception cannot understand light and color in the same way as a person with normal eyesight. However, based on models, worded explanations, physics formulae, discussions about hues, brightness, blends, and fashions, the person can certainly communicate concepts of color that those with sight can relate to based on their experiences that included visual input. Further, even though specific aspects of color may have no personal meaning, the person without sight can perform such tasks as dressing in color coordinated clothing, asking if the light is red or green before crossing streets, and other issues accepted and even demanded by society. Nuances such as emotional connotations can also be learned by those without direct experience with colors.

How the brain perceives and interprets signals from other senses to accomplish the concept formations without input from the senses it is missing is not clear. However, it is known that areas of the brain usually used as projection areas for the sense of sight can become projection areas for touch or presumably other senses. Use of a sense apparently does not increase the sensitivity of the receptor organ but seems to capture and store more signals the more the sense is used. When projection areas are not being used, the need for connections is transferred to these areas. A map of the human brain shows many areas where processes related to vision take place.

The process of adaptation to sight loss is highly individualized. Factors such as age of onset, cause of blindness, extent of loss, attitudes held toward being blind, previous learning experiences, physical health, and presence of other impairments or disabilities have impact on an individual's ability to accommodate or compensate for the lack of sight. The great impact of sight loss can increase geometrically when additional senses such as hearing loss are present. When an additional sense is lost, the same assumptions about the effects of blindness should not be made. The person then must learn and be taught in ways that take advantage of remaining senses whatever they may be.

Perhaps the most important aspect of education and rehabilitation of the blind and those with low vision is to provide the opportunities necessary to develop remaining senses and provide experiences that allow the sensations to be used in perception and concept formation.

As stated in later chapters, views about blindness held by workers for the blind as well as the blind themselves range from beliefs that all blind people are helpless to believing that lack of sight is merely a nuisance. The model presented here suggests that certain functions are lost when the sense of sight is absent. However, when the individual has sufficient time, experience, and learning opportunities, the effects of blindness can be greatly reduced and allow the person to live a productive and contented life equal to that of others in society.

DISCUSSION

This chapter is an introduction to the processes of developing perceptions. Because of the importance of the sense of sight, the anatomy, and physiology of the eye have been noted. The information was specifically geared to prepare the reader for discussions which deal with these concepts in other chapters. The authors have tried to raise questions to answer as readers go through other chapters, e.g., "what happens when the sense of sight is not available to the student or client?"

When readers look at the many other sensory channels through which humans can learn, it makes the education of children and adults with visual handicaps more optimistic and helps to explain how children and adults who have lost one of the most important senses are able to function so well. It should also help focus attention on those aspects of the educational and rehabilitation experiences which are most helpful to children and clients and areas in which they are in most need of help.

SUGGESTED READINGS

1. Gregory, R. L. (1997). *The eye and brain: The psychology of seeing.* (5th ed.). Princeton, NJ: Princeton University Press.

Chapter 9

VISION AND MOTIVATION

INTRODUCTION

Motivation is an explicit component in most learning theories, and an implicit component in all others. This is because learning and motivation are interwoven concepts. If the client or student is not motivated, very little learning takes place.

Two broad approaches are used to explain the sources of motivation in learning and motivational theories, external motivators, and internal motivators. External motivators are usually viewed as positive–rewards, or negative–punishments. Internal motivators are more complicated but can generally be classified as physiological or psychological. Each of these can be further subdivided as can the external motivators.

The reasons people act or behave in the ways they do have been the focus of philosophers for all of recorded history. Psychology itself grew out of philosophy and brought with it concerns about motivation.

Like most disciplines, philosophy, psychology, and theories about motivation experienced a "paradigm shift" at the start of the nineteenth century. Prior to that time, actions were attributed to moral tendencies within the individual for which he or she was morally responsible. In this light, people were motivated toward good because it was the "right" thing to do. If they acted in the "wrong" way it was because of a flaw in their character. Many people today still think in those terms based to a great extent on Biblical interpretations of life.

With the paradigm shift over the past two centuries, many thinkers began to see motivation as outside forces acting upon the individual over which he or she had little or no control. Most theories tended to see the individual as the passive recipient of these forces, both internal in the form of instincts and biological drives or from the external world in terms of social demands and the physical environment of the world.

Dr. Neal Flinders has supported the move toward more extensive belief in the external motivation paradigm shift in terms of his "bottle theory." He indicates that many aspects of life are viewed in terms of content, process, and product. If you want to make a car, you would have to have the materials or parts, which would be put together according to a planned process, and the outcome, hopefully, would be an automobile. Dr. Flinders argues that this paradigm is missing an important component: the context. For example, if you want to build a ship within a bottle, you will be constrained by the size of the bottle as you select the materials, the tools you use in the construction process and the size of the final product. Thus, the time place and circumstance are major external sources of motivation.

In a like manner, the theories used in education and psychology are constrained by the world view and the sociocultural milieu in which they exist. The scientific outlook that prevails in the physical sciences is partly responsible for this, but the influence for change is much broader than that. From the religious orientation which characterized the founding of this country, there has been a shift to a secular orientation with a strong undercurrent of materialistic reductionism as noted in an earlier chapter.

Society as a whole has not adopted the secular orientation, though it is growing in acceptance. Opinion polls, however, indicate that a large majority of individual citizens still hold to a religious orientation. The emphasis on cultural pluralism makes it possible for these two orientations to exist side by side without much overt conflict except at certain friction points such as schools, where creation and evolution as well as specific dogma are challenged; or, in civic affairs where the role of church and state are uncertain. Present lawsuits challenging prayers at commencement exercises and in classrooms are examples. Another friction point is the "pro-life pro-abortion" conflict. It appears that the entire judicial system has largely adopted the secular orientation. In like manner, the rehabilitative and educational systems have yielded to the secularist pressure or have been forced to adopt this position by court decisions.

In the selection of an intellectual frame-of-reference, one is free to use whatever theories or model that seem most likely to produce positive change. As noted in Chapter 5, scientists do not have consensus in criteria for evaluating assumptions in science. Likewise, In motivational theories, people are free to choose from among the theories available and the assumptions upon which they rest. It is important for professionals to understand the basis of motivation and select one or a blend of theories when presenting services in order to engage the student/client in the education or training process.

This chapter will review several of the most popular motivational theories and consider research evidence in support of these. The intent is to provide professionals with choices that can guide their rehabilitative and educational practices as they work with children and adults with visual disabilities.

OBJECTIVES

Upon completion of this chapter the reader will be able to:

1. Describe several motivational theories and the assumptions upon which they are founded.
2. Make a tentative choice from among several theories for the approaches to be used in completing professional duties, and understand the consequences which follow from the particular theories chosen.
3. Evaluate theories of motivation for their contributions toward understanding the growth and development of people with visual handicaps as they progress through life.
4. Relate motivational theories to such issues as self-concept, self-esteem, attitude formation and modifications in the area of vision loss.

MEANING OF MOTIVATION

The original meaning of the term "motive" was to move. The reasons why an individual or organism moves or acts of its own volitions (arousal) and the goals or ends of such actions (incentives) have become included in the present meaning of the term. The notion of motivation is based on the assumption that whatever acts is "caused" to move, i.e., that actions do not occur without some "push" or "pull." The following analogy will illustrate.

An automobile will not move unless energy is supplied. Some energy, preferably in the form of the combustion of gasoline, is necessary. If this energy is not provided, the car does not move. Whether viewed as internal or external motivation, humans require a push fueled by energy just like machines.

The automobile must also be steered toward a destination or goal. The automobile does not supply on its own either the energy to get it moving or the direction of its movement. It is acted upon from without.

Human and animal motivation is often viewed in the same way. Humans are seen as material entities which are motivated by energy systems impinging upon them. The goal or direction of action must also be accounted for in terms of externally-imposed incentives.

A few modern theories are moving toward a renewal of this approach—particularly "agentive" psychology—but most psychologists remain within the framework of the nonpurposive behaviors arising from the very being of the individual.

Typically, clients are seen as acting or behaving because they are acted upon unless the assumption that the individual has the ability to generate goals independent from the outside influences. The teacher or family is seen as the supplier of these actions. They (teachers and family) are also seen as being acted upon by still other actors. Presumably, one could trace an endless chain of cause-and-effect relationships back to some original "first cause." In some instances, this might be the hypothesized "big bang" which presumably started the universe or in a religious view the first cause could be viewed as a supreme being or power.

Some moderns vary this picture by suggesting that a "causal chain" is too rigid and deterministic and that action sequences are based on probability, with chance factors influencing actions in a random or chaotic fashion. When the client is "reduced" to his/her physical properties—with soul, spirit, mind, intellect removed from the picture or redefined to physical correlates—then one has a difficult time avoiding the necessary reasoning of the modern paradigm.

Most motivational theories are based upon the above-described models: instinct theory, which grew out of Darwin's theory of evolution; drive-reduction theory, which was based on a combination of biology and behaviorism; needs theory, which was a combination of biology and social psychology; competence theory, which was based on social psychology and observations of children during development; and cognitive-balance theory, which was based on naturalistic research of people who were observed in actual settings. These will be elaborated on here.

In the "prebottle paradigm" (before Neil Flinders suggested that motivations depended on content, process, and outcomes), both the energy and goals were assumed to be within the individual and constitute the essence of life activities. A theory that is based on the preparadigm change model is "agentive theory." This approach holds that human beings are, by nature, able to make decisions and choices which are not traceable to either biological or environmental antecedents. It leaves largely unanswered questions about the origin of this ability, but it is assumed that these powers are resident within the individual.

Since human beings are able to make actual and unpredictable choices, they are responsible for their own actions. Others believe that even some of these choices and actions can be influenced by both biological and social factors. For example, Dr. Alan Bergen has observed that psychologists cannot account for more than 30 percent to 40 percent of the variance in any major human outcome no matter how many potential variables are used in the statistical models. The 60 percent to 70 percent of the variance is usually attributed to errors of measurement. Dr. Bergan maintains that this is inappropriate and agency is a better explanation. Such outcomes as success in school, marriage, employment, etc. defy standard scientific methods for determining cause-and-effect relationships. It should be noted that there is some strong supporting empirical evidence for a relationship between perceived control of one's actions whether it is real or not.

Locus-of-control studies have shown a strong relationship between an internal-locus-of-control and achievement in school and other settings. Even if this perceived control is an illusion, it is still powerfully influential in predicting human outcomes. If educators and rehabilitation specialists (including teachers and rehabilitation workers of the visually impaired) can persuade clients that they are responsible for what they learn in school, academic, social, and employment outcomes will be more positive. How lack of sight changes the impact of internal and external motivators will be discussed next.

Before research studies can be conducted which bear on factors besides cognitive, affective, and behavioral variables which may hold promise for increasing the ability to be more effective teachers, there must be an expansion of the vision of what variables are important parts of motivation, such as conative, axiology, and teleology. These three variables that were once standard fare in psychology but have been discarded with the paradigm shift are the study of volition or will or conative processes; study of values or axiology; and study of purpose, intent, or teleological variables. One could study conative processes by looking at how individuals make choices and decisions. It can be trained by encouraging clients to make choices and then allowing them to experience the consequences of those choices. Axiological studies could be conducted by comparing choices made under specified conditions such as when the subject is stressed. And, teleological studies would involve observing the persistence and energy expenditure as clients make decisions and embark on their implementation.

It would seem that researchers who have grown up with current behaviorist philosophies do not regard the absence of these variables in studies of motivation as important for today's world. However, since those without sight must rely more heavily on internal concept formation, it would be interesting to see how important these variable are for them.

Observers have noticed that blind children seem to lack "normal' motivation. Perhaps lack of sight impacts the internal formation of values and decision-making and accounts for these observations. Thorough study of these issues is beyond the scope of this discussion but is fertile ground for further investigation.

EFFECTS OF SIGHT LOSS ON MOTIVATION

Little research has been conducted with respect to motivational factors in the visually impaired. However, observations by Frailer and Warren note that young children who are blind reach for objects later than their peers with normal sight. It is suggested that reaching using sound simply occurs later than reaching based on sight.

One can speculate that a child who sees and moves toward objects is rewarded by obtaining them more often than a child without sight who hears and moves toward the object. One reason to think this is that visual form of a distant object is more likely to stay constant than sound if sound is present at all. If the sound ceases or changes intensity due to movements, it may change the intensity or vary the ability of the sound to attract the child in other ways. It may be that it takes more focus of attention to renew the attraction or that sound simply is not as motivating. Regardless of the cause, it seems clear that lack of vision has some delaying effects on a blind child's efforts to explore. Fear of moving into the unknown may also demotivate the child.

Another component of motivation discussed by White is the feeling of competence when one "knows" that he or she can do significant tasks. Many common tasks may take longer for a person who is blind to accomplish simply because tactile scanning is slower than visual scanning. Often, those who work with blind children and adults eliminate the motivating force of competence by doing too much for the blind person. This learned helplessness sometimes discussed by professionals stems from students' or adults' being deprived of motivation that comes from an internal pride in achievement.

A subcomponent of competence is competition. Academics, employment, and many forms of recreation depend on completing a task in a given amount of time. As discussed above, many tasks simply take more time for a person who is blind or who has limited visions to accomplish. The lack of success in competitive situations that are beyond the control of the person who is blind demotivate. It is essential to use teaching techniques that "level the playing field" but maintain the sense of achievement. The success in performance of tasks of equal value to those performed by sighted individuals is a major way to gain an internal sense of competence and increase motivation toward further success. Parents, teachers, counselors, and other professionals should guard against depriving children, students, and clients of a feeling of competence. It was indicated earlier in this chapter that prevalent motivation theories favor the idea that motivation comes from outside the individual. Here again it would seem that this viewpoint does not account for motivation in those who are blind or visually impaired. Ferrell, in her assessment chapter in "Education of the Visually Handicapped," notes that use of standard reinforcement procedures creates the "good fairy" syndrome in blind children because they are not able to recognize the connection between their own behaviors and the rewards they receive. If a contingency-management procedure is to be used with visually-impaired children, it seems appropriate to plan for explicit rewards for clearly-defined tasks.

Most of the outcomes observed with reinforcement procedures can be explained in terms of cognitive theory. For example, there are essentially three types of reinforcement schedules:

1. Fixed-ratio reinforcements in which a reward is given for a specified number of actions as in piece-work in a factory.
2. Fixed interval schedules in which a reinforcement is given if the behavior occurs at least a minimum number of times during a specified time period. This is like bureaucratic employment in which the worker must be present to punch the time clock and perform some minimum amount of work, but the pay is not connected to output.
3. Variable-ratio or variable-interval reinforcement. In this approach, the subject is not able to anticipate exactly when the reinforcement will occur, but experience has taught that it will come if the behavior is emitted long enough. This is a gambling approach in which the slot-machine is operated over and over again with the expectation that eventually there will be a jackpot.

Fixed-ratio schedules are very useful in establishing a behavior, but as soon as the reinforcements are withdrawn, the behaviors may cease in a short period of time. The variable schedule, once a behavior is established, is good for maintaining a behavior over long periods of time.

Behavioral theory has a difficult time explaining this phenomenon, but if the cognitive theory is applied, the effects of different schedules of reinforcement can be explained in terms of subject expectations, with reinforcements interpreted as feedback for actions taken. Even the anticipation of punishments in deterring behaviors can be explained in terms of risk anticipation or expectancy. In other words, the involvement of the learner as an active participant improves prospects for change-learning when compared with the consideration of the subject as a passive victim of reward or punishment-giving. Contingency reinforcement is widely used in classrooms and in many adult training settings. It is a very useful education technology but is not as effective unless coupled with internal factors of motivation.

As suggested earlier, one aspect of outside motivation is social interaction. Much of our social behavior is shaped by visual feedback from "body language" and observation of behavior modeled by others. Most of these essential sources of social information are only observable through the sense of sight. Those without sight often lack facial expression, engage in repetitive rocking, light filtering, and other "blindisms," dress inappropriately, and lack personal care. These are socially limiting behaviors. Many times, these behaviors are due to lack of social pressure that would normally be communicated to an individual by the general public through nonverbal means that are not seen by the person with visual impairments. A blind person has the same needs for social acceptance but will not be motivated by social customs and mores unless made aware of them in specific ways. This is another area of life in which persons who are blind may be judged to lack motivation because they do not conform to or seem to care if they conform to social actions.

Human actions are so complex and variable that no one theory has yet been developed which accounts for all of them. Perhaps the popularity of the Maslow hierarchy-of-needs approach stems from its attempt to provide a variety of need levels which recognizes that no one approach is adequate. Any approach which claims to account for all human motives should be viewed with suspicion.

The highest level of need attainment in Maslow's model is self-actualization. Most educators believe that this is a very useful concept, but it still appears to be selfish in nature. There are individuals who are willing to commit their time and energy to a cause without thought of reward attainment, punishment avoidance, or even guilt soothing motives. Rather, the "cause" is the important thing, even if it requires the sacrifice of self in the process of moving toward its realization. This level of commitment is indeed rare, but it must be accounted for in any theory of motivation. Only when values, choice, and purpose are included as constructs in a theory of motivation, it seems, can this be explained and predicted.

DISCUSSION

It should be obvious that motivation is much too complex a process to be fully developed in a single chapter. This written presentation provides an overview of the topic. It has also attempted to provide some insight into how lack of sight demotivates through reducing intrinsic and extrinsic forms of motivation that play important roles in achievement of those with normal sight.

It is hoped that readers will continue to study motivation, even perhaps conduct experiments, and endeavor to find ways in which visually-impaired children and adults can be taught that strengthens their motivation to achieve their personal goals. The authors are not attempting to impose a particular approach, but rather to sensitize readers to some of the issues involved.

The next chapter will extend the discussion of motivation to include an aspect of psychology which is beginning to be recognized as an important variable, i.e., emotions. Emotions combine subjective feelings with overt expressions which serve many functions in adapting to life's challenges.

SUGGESTED READINGS

1. Ferrell, K.A. (1985). *Reach out and teach.* New York: American Foundation for the Blind.
2. Flinders, N. (1990). *Teach the children: An agency approach to education.* Provo, UT: Mormon Research Foundation.
3. Fraiberg, S., Siegel, B., & Gibson, R. (1966). The role of sound in the search behavior of a blind infant. *Psychoanalytic Study of the Child, 21,* 327–357.
4. Scholl, G.T. (1986). *Foundations of education for blind and visually handicapped children and youth: Theory and practice.* New York: American Foundation for the Blind.
5. White, R. (1959). Motivation reconsidered: The concept of competence. *Psychological Review, 66*(5):297–333.

Chapter 10

VISION AND EMOTION

INTRODUCTION

The term "emotion" is derived from the same root as motivation—"mover" which means to move plus "ex," which means "out." So, emotion means "to move out." It represents the "arousal" component of motivation. Like motivation, emotions have been the topic of much thought and research for centuries. Before the change in world view mentioned in the last chapter, the spirit, mind, or soul was considered the source of emotional reactions. Such expressions as "moved by the spirit," which are still a part of contemporary language, reflect that earlier concept. Other expressions from this earlier period are "passions," "feelings," and "splenetic," with the latter reflecting the notion that emotions are produced by "humors" produced by specific body organs.

Scientific research and observations describe emotions as arising from neurochemical and neuromuscular processes. A researcher named Duschene, over a century ago, demonstrated that the facial expressions associated with various emotions could be produced reflexively by stimulating specific facial muscle groups. Even though no emotions were being expressed, these stimulated facial muscles bore strong resemblances to such emotions as joy, horror, pain, and contentment.

Emotions are generally classified into one of two groups, positive or pleasant emotions and negative or unpleasant emotions. The term "affect," used either as a noun or as an adjective, is used to designate either group.

This chapter will cover some of the theories which have been developed to account for this aspect of psychology. It is hoped that these theories will assist in better understanding this phenomenon, especially how emotions effect education and personal adjustment to the world.

OBJECTIVES

Upon completion of this chapter the reader will be able to:

1. Describe in general terms the ways in which emotions can be classified.
2. Recognize sources of emotions and their relationship to normal human psychological processes in children and in adult human beings.
3. Select and develop rehabilitative and educational approaches which will use both positive and negative emotions in achieving positive mental health.
4. Recognize mild emotional disturbances arising from rehabilitative and educational processes in visually-impaired children and adults, both in and out of structured experienced.

SOURCES OF EMOTIONS

In the 1860s, Charles Darwin wrote a book entitled *The Expression of the Emotions in Animals and Men*, which is still available in many libraries. He concluded from his research, both with animals and with humans in many different cultures, that emotions are largely reflexive. There are specific kinds of stimuli which will elicit an emotional response which is expressed in changes in actions and attitudes. For example, fear will produce either immediate flight from a dangerous situation or, in stronger fear, inability to move at all. The pupils of the eye restrict, breathing quickens, and adrenal hormones are released into the blood stream.

On the positive side, smiling is universally recognized as a sign of a pleasant feeling. It is usually accompanied with relaxed muscles, slowed breathing, and dilation of the pupils in the eye. The smiling response is observed in infants during the first few months of life. It is elicited by a human face in motion, or (as in the case of a blind infant) by a human voice. Learning does not appear to play any part in this early expression.

Hebb and Thompson, in their article, "The Significance of Animal Studies for Social Psychology," cite evidence that emotions are highly correlated with intelligence. They claim that both the number of emotions and the variety of stimuli which evoke them increase as one moves up both the phyletic (a classification of animals along an evolutionary hierarchy) scale and the "onto genetic" (development within a single species) scale. These changes along the scale are also associated with increased intelligence. Their compelling discussion leads one to wonder whether emotions are primarily increased sensitivities to the world in which an individual lives and how they provide assistance in the adaptation to the world.

Their hypothesis that societies, although not creating or teaching emotions, try to influence the ways in which emotions are expressed and in controlling exposure to negatively arousing stimuli is an excellent summary of numerous research studies which bear on these issues. It would help explain why those with physical disabilities or unusual or unexpected characteristics are treated differently than those from one's particular social group.

The hypothesis also provides a basis for understanding emotional disturbance in individuals. One can be unable to keep one's reactions to emotionally disturbing stimuli within socially prescribed bounds. This could be the result of ignorance of the standards, lack of previous experience with the aroused emotions, or overexposure to arousing patterns of stimuli.

A treatment program could be built around these factors which would look at basic causes rather than focusing on evoked behaviors alone. For example, treatment would be geared toward learning to control the stimuli which evoke a fear response rather than on modifying the fear behavior itself. As one reads this chapter, he/she should think about other possible applications in rehabilitative and educational programs with visually impaired persons.

SOCIETY'S EMOTIONAL REACTION

One of the major reasons for studying emotions in this book is the observation that blindness, either in thought or observation, arouses a variety of emotions in sighted and blind persons. To some extent, these emotions are mediated by a person's culture. For example, an old Hindu proverb says: "When you see a blind man, kick him. Why should you be kinder to him than his gods have been?" In contrast, the Judeo-Christian view is that the blind should be pitied and protected, and should allow others to show forth God's will by offering assistance, even as Jesus did, to blind individuals.

Perhaps neither view represents a valuable guide for working with those with vision loss. In the former case, a bad situation would be made even worse. In the latter, if too much help is given, the blind person may be denied the opportunity to develop his/her natural talents for his/her personal benefit and to the betterment of society.

FREUD'S EXPLORATION OF EMOTIONS

Modern explorations of emotions began with papers written by Sigmund Freud. Freud's legacy tends to view emotions as negative, and, by definition, irrational. He viewed the Id as the source of an instinctive energy, termed Libido or life-seeking force, which always seeks the pleasurable. There are specific things which will satisfy the Id but it is essentially blind to other than primal needs. The Ego develops out of the Id, but is affected by patterns of nurturing. It develops the ability to see things as they really are, and are essentially rational.

Although there is virtually no research supporting Freud's theory, it still has wide currency in the Western culture. Perhaps this is because he was an excellent writer, he was first to set down his ideas clearly, and his ideas are quite simple to understand. Freud's ideas became the basis for much of later concepts including the importance of emotions. Since Freud's time, many have proposed models to help understand how emotions influence behavior and attitudes.

ROBERT PLUTCHIK'S THEORY OF EMOTIONS

An example of models to explain how emotions work is charts which classify human emotions found in the book by Robert Plutchik entitled simply *Emotions*. The illustration is described as follows: if one were to cut a sphere in half through its poles, one hemisphere would represent negative emotions and the other positive emotions. Around the equator are listed the emotions, with each emotion's opposite located 180 degrees away. As one moves from the equator toward the poles, one would find greater intensities of emotions.

As one moves from the equator toward the poles, he/she should note that the number of emotions is surprisingly large. The English language is not well suited to the description of emotions. People certainly have great difficulty in trying to describe how they feel and verbally express emotions. Some languages have many words to express the concept of a single emotion such as love, hate, etc. And, many terms such as the Spanish term "simpatico" have no comparable term for translation into English. Perhaps Plutchik's taxonomy could be used to enrich the expressions of emotion.

Emotions can be aroused by either actual or perceived situations. Falling or unexpected flashes of light are sources of the basic emotion of fear in young infants and elicit the physical changes that occur with fear described earlier. The basic emotion of fear may be tempered through experience and practice as we become adults. However, even when one is comfortably seated in a theater and viewing a movie, actions on the screen can cause the same emotional response to illusions produced by the camera as an actual experience.

Many words also are emotionally "loaded," i.e., they arouse emotions. Some responses to particular words occur because of past experience, but many have power to cause changes in our emotional state because of the values which the society in which one lives attributes to them. Media advertising is an example of the use of "emotive" words. Words such as first, love, new, and free are used liberally in advertising to get our attention and move us to buy products or services. Likewise, pictures with sexual meaning, including masculine or feminine attractiveness, are used to entice us to buy products or participate in activities.

Like the model described above, each of the positive emotionally laden terms has its opposite. Such opposing words can be used to discredit or devalue thoughts, concepts, and even people. Words such as ugly, expensive, black, or dumb are sometimes used in derogatory fashions.

BLINDNESS AND EMOTIONS

The word "blind," referring to blindness, is an emotionally charged word. It most often elicits emotions of fear or pity in people, though most have had no actual experience of being blind or even a close association with someone who is blind. Studies have shown that of serious health conditions one might encounter, blindness is usually ranked near cancer as most dreaded.

Perhaps the reason for the fear evoked when considering being blind is because those who have grown up with sight cannot imagine how they would perform without sight. Also, many individuals, as children, played "Blind Man's Bluff" and felt foolish because they could not do even simple tasks when blindfolded. Regardless of the cause, our society as a whole has very strong feelings about blindness and people who are blind.

Those who are blind, or work as educators and rehabilitation specialists, should take time to analyze their reactions to being blind. Hopefully, each person can come to a useful understanding of blindness and not let the common emotional responses of fear or pity or unfounded admiration interfere with social interactions or reduce access to success for individuals who are blind or have low vision. There are several viewpoints which professionals should consider and understand.

The book *A Psychiatrist Looks at Blindness* by Cholden is based on Freud's theory. In brief, the concepts in this book uses a psychoanalytic concept that before a person who loses his/her sight can be rehabilitated, he/she must stop viewing him/herself as a sighted person and start viewing him/herself as a blind person. This requires the person to look deeply into his or her own feelings and recognize him/herself, as a blind person with self-worth and who is competent. Stated another way, the person is reborn as a person without sight. Further, Cholden's concept holds that the problems associated with training and rehabilitation of those with blindness are caused by an internal perspective, and if that can be changed to a positive image, chances of rehabilitation and education are greatly improved. Being blind himself, Cholden presents some interesting insights, but for the most part, they should be considered as speculations needing research support, rather than as valid truths.

A second viewpoint is that being blind or having low vision is a mere nuisance that need not impact the life of the individual. In this view, each individual is challenged to overcome any obstacle that prevents "normal" activities through his own effort. Those who espouse this view use examples of outstanding success by individuals who are blind to banish any negative, emotionally charged concepts about being blind. In some rehabilitation and education programs, if the person who is blind does not succeed, the blame is placed on society's lack of acceptance. In other words, disabilities caused by lack of sight are discounted and barriers to success are external to the individual. The conclusion is that if society's feelings related to blindness can be changed, then chances of rehabilitation are improved. Training using these tenets encourages the use of aggressive confrontation of perceived barriers to success.

A third view is proposed by Dean Tuttle in his book, *Self-Esteem and Adjusting with Blindness*. In this discussion, the individual self-worth is maintained by adjusting with blindness (a disability) and overcoming the challenges faced by those without sight. Many challenges are real to a blind person, such as: access to information in accessible formats, freedom of travel, attitudinal barriers to employment, etc. Success requires maintaining and/or developing strong self-esteem. This is accomplished by gaining skills which allow the individual without sight to function within the community in which he or she chooses to live. This approach to success requires a building of self-esteem by gaining an internal sense of competence and adjustment to the real limitations imposed by society and the physical settings in which people who are blind find themselves.

Professionals and organizations that provide services to the blind operate on one or a combination of these emotionally generated belief systems. Often the internally-based or externally-based philosophies which underlie their choices of service have not been examined. Yet, the attitudes that children or adults have when completing the program may have been passed along unconsciously based on emotions from one of these sources rather than chosen after due consideration.

In addition, professionals who serve individuals who are blind or have low vision need to consider the source and consequences of emotions felt in reaction to the word blind. Those who come from experiences that view blindness as only a personal/internal problem may blame themselves for lack of success because they cannot accept their state. Those whose experiences treat blindness as a nuisance may become frustrated because they feel others are not giving them a "fair shake." Their thoughts include, "I am OK, but, I am not as successful as I would like. So, it must be an external reason for my lack of success."

Organizations or individuals who are driven by extreme internal or external sources of emotions will not likely be viewed in a realistic way or be effective in the process of understanding the effects and affects caused by being blind. Some examples of the effects of emotion in the models cited above are as follows.

If the student or client who is blind is viewed as having trouble accepting his blindness, i.e., seeing himself as a blind person then his or her efforts may not be driven by the need to seek solutions to real problems because there is hope of gaining sight or finding other ways to maintain the current self-image. The result is the person seems passive and becomes the object of frustration or pity by those who try to help or by those with whom they associate.

On the other hand, if a student or client is viewed or taught that blindness does not have a significant impact, then he or she may begin to look for outside-of-self reasons for his or her frustrations. In order to maintain a high self-esteem, an individual who is blind or who has low vision may blame others or some outside circumstance when personal characteristics or unrealistic assessments of skills are the source for lack of success.

DISCUSSION

Personal emotions play an important role in all of people's lives. Perhaps everyone should seek for a theory of emotions which will allow them to see more clearly what they are and how they influence efforts to be effective human beings. (Incidentally, the Greek word from which the English term "theory" is derived, means "to see clearly".) It is hoped that the discussion here makes it clear how emotionally charged work for the blind is and that professionals and blind persons themselves will evaluate their reactions to blindness and/or being blind.

Emotions provide a bridge between the concepts of motivation and the topic of our next chapter: attitudes. As noted above, one view of emotions is that they provide the "arousal" component in motivation. Attitudes, in part, can provide persons with the "cue" or "incentive" component of motivation. The "positive" and "negative" aspects of attitudes are strongly related to positive and negative emotions.

SUGGESTED READINGS

1. Plutchik, R. (1980). *Emotions, a psychoevolutionary synthesis.* New York: Harper & Row.
2. Hebb, D.O., & Thompson, W.R. (1954). The social significance of animal studies In G. Lindsay & E. Arouson (eds.), *The handbook of social psychology,* vol. 2 (2d ed.). Boston: Addison-Wesley, 729–774.
3. Cholden, L.S. *A psychiatrist works with blindness.* New York: American Foundation for the Blind.
4. Tuttle, D. (2004). *Self-esteem and adjusting with blindness* (3rd ed.). Springfield, IL: Charles C Thomas.

Chapter 11

VISION AND ATTITUDES

INTRODUCTION

In the 1950s and 1960s, there was much interest in the concept of "attitudes." Attitudes were defined in many ways, but the standard dictionary definition was: "Attitudes are a posturing of the mind in preparation for action; a behavioral predisposition." People have attitudes toward virtually everything about which they have an awareness, whether objects, events, or persons. They can be positive, negative, or neutral in valance, and they can be high or low in intensity.

Interest faded in the study of attitudes primarily because: (1) behavioral theory has dominated psychology for the last decades, and it emphasizes overt behavior rather than internal processes which influence actions including attitudes; and (2) because of the difficulties in measuring directly the attitudes people possess. In recent years, a renewal of interest in attitude theory and measurement has arisen as behavioral influence has waned and cognitive theories have reemerged as important contributors in education and psychology.

The above-mentioned trends have been particularly true of attitude studies concerning blindness and vision loss: both public attitudes held toward the blind and attitudes which the blind themselves hold toward their condition. And, although attitudes are still difficult to measure, newer ideas and technology have offered hope for being able to measure them.

This chapter will first look at attitude theory. Next it will consider research concerning attitudes toward the disabled. This will be followed by a discussion of attitudes toward the blind, and with suggestions for using this theory in rehabilitative and educational programs with the visually impaired.

OBJECTIVES

Upon completion of this chapter the reader will be able to:

1. Define attitudes in terms of the three components of an attitude: behavioral, affective, and cognitive.
2. Describe methods used in the measurement of attitudes, including social-distance scales, Likert scales, and Thurston successive-interval scales.
3. Recognize the dimensions along which attitudes toward different groups differ and their use in comparing groups of disabled children.
4. Use attitude theory as a means of understanding better the problems of the visually impaired in education, employment, and full participation in the "mainstream" of society.

COMPONENTS OF ATTITUDES

The following materials describe the components of attitudes which should help in understanding methods for changing them. Attitudes are a more specific way of viewing concepts. Both attitudes and concepts contain information or cognitive meanings, whether or not the information is correct. Both are organized in an hierarchical fashion, with superordinate, coordinate, and subordinate relationships. Also, both can be defined in terms of attributes, characteristics, properties, or qualities of exemplars which the members of a group share and which are used to define the group.

In practice, concepts and attitudes are distinguished in terms of the uses to which they are put. Concepts are used primarily in "knowing" about something, while attitudes are considered as reflecting "feelings" about something. Both concepts and attitudes contain elements or components which have been labeled as cognitive, affective, and behavioral, but the use to which they are put determines their category-as a concept or as an attitude.

For example, one might know a great deal about icebergs, but not have much by way of feelings or actions to be observed with respect to them. On the other hand, if a person has lost a family member in the sinking of a ship which came in contact with an iceberg, that person still does not know much about icebergs, but he/she will have strong feelings associated with them. One might have fears, express hate, or feel disgust when icebergs are mentioned in a conversation. One might also have strong behavioral predispositions toward icebergs, e.g., one would want to act in order to stay as far from them as possible. In the first instance, a concept-classification approach would seem most appropriate, while in the latter, it would be best to classify them as attitudes.

In the course of cognitive development, people come in contact with many aspects of the world, and they structure these contacts in the form of concepts. Some of these contacts will engender little or nothing more than dispassionate, intellectual experiences. Other contacts will create feelings, either positive or negative, but with very little intellectual content. Still other contacts will move to actions, but contain little intellectual or feeling reactions. In most instances, however, all three components will be developed, but not in the same amount or to the same level.

NEGATIVE ATTITUDES

There is a widely held notion that people have negative attitudes or prejudices only toward those things in their lives which they know relatively little about. They tend to be "down on what they are not up on." There is a measure of validity for this idea in the notion of "xenophobia" or fear of the strange or fear of strangers. On the other hand, there seems to be a strong interest and attraction to the new or novel, in the anticipation of an experience one has never had before; for example, thrill rides at amusement parks or "scary" movies. In either case, the fear or anticipation seems to be measured against a backdrop of the known or familiar. And, if new ideas are presented in a boring way, it may engender neither fear nor anticipation. In short, the new is not in itself able to account for the feeling component in attitudes.

As noted in the last chapter, Hebb and Thompson cite evidence that emotions are triggered when people are exposed to a specific set of stimuli within a specific context. For example, an adult with little prior experience with snakes, will show fear or disgust when exposed to them. The response will be less pronounced if the exposure takes place within a safe environment such as a zoo in which the snake is confined behind a glass window in contrast to being exposed as they run into a snake on the kitchen table. On the positive side, tiny infants smile at the face of their mother but will show fear of a strange face after the age of six months. The past experience of the person with the specific stimuli influences whether the response is positive or negative.

Allport and Kramer, in discussing the origins of prejudice, suggest that some people may remember dangerous encounters with a particular racial group which never occurred. They cite no evidence that this is the case, but, real or imagined, the prior experience is important.

Work has been done with a process called "desensitization," in which one is exposed gradually to a stimulus which originally produced an emotional response, but in a nonthreatening milieu. It may well be that the favorableness or unfavorableness of attitudes must be considered in terms of overall experiences and that generalizations are difficult or dangerous to make.

The study of racial, ethnic, and/or minority-group prejudice (negative attitudes) has been complicated by the political, legal, and social climate of our nation. Laws are passed which attempt to control conduct toward certain groups of people with the expectation that attitudes will become more positive with these controlled behaviors. Racial prejudice will diminish as school children are integrated into racially-balanced classrooms. Ethnic barriers will be removed if all families are forced to live in the same neighborhoods as neighbors. The young will automatically love and respect the elderly by bringing them together in shared activities.

Although laws may control, under coercive threats, overt actions, there is little evidence that basic, underlying feelings have been changed. There is as much opposition to racial integration in the schools today as in the days before *Brown v. Board of Education* in 1954. The feelings are simply not expressed overtly. The roots of prejudice have not been generally recognized or addressed adequately.

ATTITUDES TOWARD THE DISABLED

There is some evidence that it is the quality of the experiences which people have with these groups rather than the quantity of contacts which influence negative attitudes toward the positive. For example, in racial school integration, children of both Black and Caucasian backgrounds in the average and below-average economic strata of society show increased prejudice, while those who are above-average find mutually-satisfying and pleasant interactions. Disabled clients who perform at a normal or above-normal level tend to be viewed more positively by their nondisabled peers, while those who are seen as performing at a below-normal level, without any compensating contributions, are disliked. To put it another way, "physical" integration will not by itself ensure "rehabilitative and educational" or "social" integration. The overall quality of the rehabilitative and educational experience must be considered and planned for if minority groups such as the disabled are to be fully participating members of a classroom or a society.

In one set of interesting studies, children in a classroom are grouped together for problem solving. Each group has a mixture of students, each of which has part of the information needed to solve the problem. Unless every member of the group is involved, the problem cannot be solved. These groups compete with one another in finding the problem solution. It has been shown that children who were originally shunned improved in group acceptance as they were brought into the problem-solving group and his/her contribution was recognized as important.

During and immediately after World War II, Roger Barker and his associates studied attitudes of nondisabled children toward the disabled. It was found that the overtly-expressed attitudes are positive, while covert feelings are negative and produce avoidance behaviors. It was also observed from a review of research literature that the disabled as a single group or as independent subgroups do not possess distinctive personality traits. Some relationships to personality attributes, however, did emerge. The length of time a person has been disabled and the severity of the disability did show a relationship with factors such as dependency, pessimism, and apprehension.

Other studies have shown that all disabled children are not viewed in the same way by the able-bodied public. Murphy found that among educators, the behaviorally disturbed and the visually impaired were least likely to be desired as members in a regular or special education classroom. Barbara Bateman, in her doctoral research, found that children's attitudes toward visually impaired children were related to the amount of direct contact with these children. Rural children with little or no direct contact with visually impaired children viewed them more negatively and unrealistically than urban children who had more contact. Her work, along with that of Murphy, could be used to support xenophobia as the source of negative attitudes toward the visually impaired. Cholden and Cutsforth, on the other hand, tend to support the idea that the blind are, in fact, different from others and these differences engender prejudice.

In the decades of the 1950s and 1960s, a group of social psychologists from Yale University conducted research which produced evidence that personality traits were significantly correlated with prejudice. Those children who possessed a "fascist" or "authoritarian" personality tended to be more prejudiced than those with a more open and "democratic" personality. It was also shown that men, on average, were more prejudiced than women.

When Lukoff and Whiteman studied attitudes of the sighted toward the blind, they found that personality traits and gender applied here as well. They did not deal with the issue of where the source of prejudice was located, though the tenor of their reports tended to suggest it came from within the sighted children themselves.

MEASUREMENT OF ATTITUDES

Many approaches have been developed for the measurement of attitudes. None has yet been capable of avoiding one major pitfall, i.e., validity. Almost all are self-reports which are very transparent to the person taking the test. Few people want to admit that they are prejudiced and so, to some extent, they will not always be completely truthful. Most attitude inventories are quite short, and it would, therefore, be difficult to include items based on the Edwards Social Desirability Scale as a part of the instrument.

A typical scale for the measurement of attitudes would consist of a series of statements. Subjects would indicate whether and to what extent they agree or disagree with each statement. For example, one could respond to the statement: "Most blind children lose their sight because of social (venereal) diseases." If one strongly agrees with this statement, they could rate it as a 5 or a 4 if they slightly agree, a 3 if they don't know, a 2 if they slightly disagree, and a 1 if they strongly disagree. The summed scores would supposedly indicate amount of prejudice.

Another approach is the Bogardus Social Distance Scale. Here, items are selected in terms of remote to intimate social relations ranging from living in the same community with the persons toward whom the attitudes are held to being married to them. The greater the number and closeness of contacts which would be tolerated would be an indication of attitudes.

To reduce some of the scaling problems in constructing such an inventory, L. L. Turnston developed his successive-interval scale. In this approach, a large number of items, typically 200 to 300 items, are developed which range from very positive, through neutral to very negative, based on the developers' judgment. These items are then presented to a large number of "judges" who assign a number to each item which reflects his/her judgment of its place on a scale. These judgments are summed, averaged, and standard-deviations determined. Those items which are seen by most judges as being at a certain point on the scale can be selected to form a relatively small number of items which will range from very positive to very negative. Test subjects, those having the attitudes, are then asked to indicate whether they agree or disagree with each statement and to indicate with a number how strongly they agree or disagree.

The work of Ekhardt Hess holds great promise for the direct measurement of attitudes by measuring the size of the subject's eye pupil when presented with a picture of the object of the inventory. The pupil will increase if the subject has positive reactions to the picture, and decrease when attitudes are negative. Hess's early work holds promise, but it is expensive and complicated. If the equipment could be updated by using video cameras and computer monitors, it could be very useful.

If a valid and reliable attitude measuring instrument were available, it could be used for:

1. Selecting personnel to work with the blind;
2. Observing changes in attitude such as before- and after-measures for a training project;
3. Measuring self-attitudes among various subgroups of visually-impaired children, etc.

This chapter is fundamental to an understanding of one of the most pervasive problems faced by minority groups. As noted at the beginning, it is designed to give the reader an overview of the psychological and social problems associated with attitudes about vision loss. The coverage, of necessity, has been superficial, but the topics should point the reader toward more detailed coverage, both in other books and for the rest of one's professional career.

SUGGESTED READINGS

1. Allport, G.W., & B.M. Kramer. (1949). Some roots of prejudice. *Journal of Psychology, 22:9–39.*
2. Barker, R.G. (1953). Adjustment to physical handicap and illness: A survey of the social psychology of physique and disability. *Social Science Research Council Bulletin, 55.*
3. Bateman, B.D. (1962). *Reading and psycholinguistic processes of partially sighted children.* Urbana-Champaign, IL: University of Illinois Press.
4. Bateman, B. (1965). Psychological evaluation of blind children. *New Outlook for the Blind, 59,* 193–196.
5. Cholden, L.S. (1958). *A psychiatrist works with blindness.* New York: American Foudation for the Blind.
6. Cutsforth, T.D. (1951). *The blind in school and society.* New York: American Foundation for the Blind.
7. Lukoff, I.F., & Whiteman, M. (1970). Socialization and segregated education. *Research Bulletin,* American Foundation for the Blind, *20,* 91–107.

Chapter 12

VISION AND SELF-CONCEPT

INTRODUCTION

In Chapter 1, of this book, concepts were defined in terms of a process which reduces the complexity of the world in which humans live. As people build up concepts–categories or groupings of objects, persons or events–it was suggested that they are organized into superordinate, coordinate, and subordinate systems, with the total representing the world view. If this conceptual system changes, so will the world view.

In the previous chapter, it was further suggested that concepts and attitudes are interchangeable for the most part. The world view, then, is the sum total of the concepts and attitudes that a person holds about the many aspects of the world he or she has experienced.

"Self-Concept" is the set of constructs and/or attitudes that one holds about and toward him/herself. This view of various aspects of personal make-up and the outlook on the world may change. Also, one is emotionally involved in the concepts he or she holds about him/herself.

Self-concepts are multiple rather than global, but they have typically been defined in terms of how one feels about various aspects of his/her person. One's body, with its various parts and systems, constitutes one aspect of "me." One's temperament, intelligence, emotional state, personality, character, gender, race, etc. are other aspects of "self" about which people have formed concepts. Other concepts are related to the relationship with aspects of the environment such as family relations, employment, citizenship, education, memberships, residence, and so forth.

Tests have been developed which measure how one feels about these various parts of one's "self." Usually, these tests consist of a series of statements which are assumed to indicate acceptance or rejection of how one feels about the various aspects of personal traits. For example, one might be asked to answer questions about the "intellectual self" that attempts to measure how one views that part of his/her make-up, i.e., do they believe they are bright, dull, average, a good student, smart, etc. His/her responses are compared with how others have answered these questions about themselves. In other words, measures of these parts of the self-concept are formed based on answers from various demographic groups so one can see how closely an individual's answers conform to some average or standard in the views of one's "selves."

This chapter, considers some of the aspects of self and how people feel about those aspects. Then it will consider measurement procedures which give some ideas about how one feels about him/herself. Lastly, it will consider the effects of vision loss on the self-concept.

OBJECTIVES

At the end of this chapter, the reader will be able to:

1. Describe the nature of the self concept as related to theoretical models.
2. Discuss some of the methods which have been developed to assist in the measurement of self concepts.
3. Analyze the effects of vision loss on the acquisition, change, and stability of self concepts, especially as these relate to normal development, education, and rehabilitation.

HOW WE VIEW OURSELVES

A recent national poll reported that more than 90 percent of U.S. women would change some aspect(s) of their body if they could. It was further reported that among models, the same was true, i.e., these beautiful "ideal" women who are admired and envied by other women, also wanted to change some aspect of their bodies. Although weight loss was a major concern, other aspects of the body such as the relative length of the body and legs, the length of the neck, bust size, foot size, overall shape, etc. were mentioned often as needing changes.

Although the above-mentioned study was conducted on women, many men would most likely want to change some aspect of their bodies—more muscle, less stomach, taller or shorter, broader shoulders and narrower hips, amount of hair, etc.

When one thinks about oneself, one usually includes the physical self as a foundational aspect of who the self is. When people are asked to describe themselves, appearance is an essential element, including height, weight, hair color, eye color, skin color, and general build. These are considered along with how one feels about the body. People tend to categorize others, as well as themselves, in terms of their physical characteristics. As an exercise in identifying the attributes which are most important to the reader, both with respect to others and to him/her self, assume that one is in college, single, and is playing the dating game. A friend has offered to "set him or her up" on a blind date. Before one accepts this offer, he or she will most likely have some questions about the prospective date. What would these questions include? Would one be concerned about age, complexion, hair and eye color, size, neatness, appearance, etc.? Other questions would most likely be included. In addition to physical characteristics other questions of concern may be asked about religion, morality, employment status, marital status, interests, shy personality or outgoing, etc. In considering the person one is about to date, should one be satisfied knowing only that the person is able to walk five steps and still be able to make steam on a cold mirror?

If one were being considered as a blind date, would one's self-concept become an issue? In other words, would one tend to classify himself/herself in the same ways one evaluates others? The answers to the above questions reflect something about the person's knowledge of the world and his/her attitudes toward it, as well as about how he or she regards himself/herself. One does not view himself/herself in isolation from one's concepts about others.

LABELING OURSELVES

In the social/cultural realm, there are many categories which are used to classify aspects of one's own nature as well as the nature of others. Some of these categorizing labels are reflected in surnames, e.g., such things as occupation—carpenter, wheelwright, sailor, farmer, etc.; titles, i.e., bishop, chamberlain, king, etc.; town of residence, e.g., Berliner, Pennfield, de la Cruz, London, etc.; physical characteristics such as short, handy, brain, etc.; specific kind of houses such as Graham (gray house), Pinkham (pink house), Grantham (grant house), etc. People also classify on the basis of relationships, nationality, temperament, and personality traits.

There are many different groups with which people identify. One can be a husband, father, brother, son, nephew, and cousin. One can also be a Mormon, a professor, faculty member, New Yorker, American, sports enthusiast, music lover, neighbor, etc. Some of these groups are further subdivided into more specific entities. For example, as a sports enthusiast, one can be a fan of the Denver Nuggets, Chicago Bears, Ohio State Buckeyes, New York Islanders, etc. Some of the groups are "networked" as in various family relationships; others are relatively independent.

As noted in Chapter 2, there are several types of attributes which are used to define the categories, e.g., criterial, functional, formal, noisy, quiet, and/or relational. Some groups with which people are associated are defined in terms of noisy attributes such as "blindness." This attribute may convey useful information, but it also creates far more emotions than understandings.

If one has been sighted, and suddenly loses sight, then this attribute will be very important for that person until an accommodation in conceptualization (a change in self-concept) is achieved. Over time, one will be less and less concerned with blindness until, in some situations, it ceases to have much meaning at all. In other situations, however, such as when meeting other people for the first time, or when one needs letters read, this quality is more important.

Again, with a person who has lost sight, as in the example just noted, one might have thought about the various groups to which she or he belongs—not in any formal way, but in the groups with which one shares identifiable attributes—there are some which are far more important than others. Students may identify a teacher as "my blind English teacher." This places far too much emphasis on the noisy attribute of blindness, and not enough emphasis on other qualities which could be considered as more descriptive of basic values. Perhaps the expression "English teacher who is blind" is a better representation of the value. Currently "person-first" descriptors of persons with disabilities is "politically" correct. Person-first phrasing is an example of trying to change both society's concept of disabilities and improve self-concepts of those with disabilities. The emphasis on the person helps increase the value of the person and improve the self-concept more.

The conceptual categories which are most important in understanding this teacher as a person would, perhaps be, first his/her adherence to Christianity as being superordinate for this person. Then might come family and profession in that order. These are the coordinate concepts which filter down to lower-order concepts. In the end, most people would rather be remembered as a friend and mentor than as a blind person.

As professionals attempt to identify the concepts which their clients hold toward themselves, as well as one's own personal self concepts, they cannot rely on tests alone to provide the necessary information. Such instruments as the *Tennessee Self Concept Scale* or the *Piers-Harris Self-Concept Test* are very useful as the professional compares one client's self concept with that of others, but they will need to help clients identify those groups with which they have the greatest affinity. Most people are reluctant to share their most personal and intimate feelings; they require a relationship of trust and mutual respect. Yet, if one understands a person's self-concept, he or she can begin to assist that person in moving toward a full and rewarding life.

In particular, the professional needs to be aware of negative self-concepts a person may hold. If a person considers himself/herself as a "nothing," it will be difficult for that person to make much progress, or to be willing to take risks in order to progress.

There is a great deal of research which shows a strong positive relationship between positive self-concept and high academic achievement. As it has been noted before, correlations do not show cause-and-effect relationships, however. During an earlier period of time, a number of research organizations attempted to increase academic achievement by improving the self-concept of students. Only one of a couple of dozen studies showed positive results. This strongly suggests that a person's self-concepts will improve as they experience success in academic and other domains. In other words, students—as well as adults—know when they are making progress toward goals, and their self-concepts will become more positive as they sense that progress is being made. A positive self-concept is more the result of, rather than the cause of, academic and other progress.

Psychologists often view blindness as one of the most devastating things which could happen, and sight restoration as about the best thing which could happen. For some people, neither of these outcomes would be as desirable as most sighted people would think. Alberto Valvo, in a study of subjects who had been without useful sight for many years, and then had surgery which restored useful sight, found that a considerable period of time—in some cases more than a year—was required before these patients were able to function as sighted persons. In other words, these patients went through the same sequence of behaviors and feelings as those losing their sight, i.e., shock, denial, anger, blaming, and, finally, acceptance. When one has developed skills which are satisfying and productive, they dislike having to learn new approaches. One could postulate that the adjustment from a state of single blessedness to marital bliss will take time and will show the same sequence as noted above. Then, with a divorce, the same sequence would be experienced again. In short, any major disruption in one's way of life will produce stress and require accommodation to the new situation and have an effect on one's self-concept.

In another context, Mary K. Bauman presented a case history of a man who had been marginal at best in his ability to hold a job and care for his family. His wife was always pushing him to function beyond his own perceived limits. After loss of sight, he was no longer expected to hold a job and provide for his family. His wife accepted this circumstance and "got off his back." He was free to sit at home, listen to talking books, and visit with his friends. His blindness was a "boon" to him rather than a great loss. It is suggested that since he was complying with new expectations, his self-concept would be improved because he viewed himself as successful in the new situation. However, it may be that as time passes, a person in this situation would soon be viewed by others as lazy or incompetent. As friends' and associates' concept of him changed, including their expectations of him and behavior toward him, his self-concept might also be affected and he may also begin to believe that he was not competent, thus lowering his self-concept.

SELF-CONCEPT AND VISION LOSS

As with other areas of measurement, there are few if any measures of self-concept which have been appropriately validated for use with individuals who are blind. At best, sometimes individuals with blindness or who have low vision have been included in the sample used to develop the measure. Studies of the self-concepts of groups who are blind typically have used samples much too small to make generalizations about such a diverse group–a group with only one characteristic in common. With limited valid measuring tools in the field of work for the blind, perhaps it is more helpful for professionals who work with those who are blind or have severe loss of sight to think about and understand how to build and maintain a positive self-concept rather than make comparisons.

If professionals can assist visually-impaired children and adults to view themselves as worthwhile and capable of learning, growing, and achieving as much as those who are sighted, they should be able to prevent many negative self-concepts from forming. And, if this is done they will help these individuals recognize that their vision loss is not so important as many sighted persons may think. Those they serve will be freed from negative attitudes about self which inhibit personal growth. As they become more and more competent, they will find that vision loss fades more and more into the background and, at least for themselves, is a far less "noisy" attribute.

Children who are blind respond to influences on self-concept in much the same way as their peers. What others believe about the abilities of a child may become a self-fulfilling prophecy. Studies in education show that when teachers believe their students are highly intelligent and "good" students, they treat them differently than if they view them as "poor" students with limited academic potential. This "halo" effect can be seen from children's earliest years. Parents must consider their view of blindness and strive to enhance their child's self-concept.

As already discussed, a self-concept is at least partially formed by how an individual is viewed and treated. As children who are blind become members of a family, it is critical that they are viewed as being more like other children than different. Unless there are disabilities in addition to blindness children who are blind can be encouraged and shown how to eat, walk, talk, play, dress, do chores, read, write, and develop social skills like their peers who are sighted. When there are no expectation and limited encouragement, children who are blind develop more slowly and are deprived of the successes which form a positive self-concept. The same is true for adults who become blind.

Parents are the most important source of feedback to children, and thus the most important source of the development of a self-concept. Those who provide early intervention and education must help parents view their child who is blind in a positive light by, if necessary, changing the parents' concept of blindness. This can be done by helping the family know adaptive techniques for teaching developmentally appropriate tasks at the ages when most children learn them. Again, this is true for families when there is an adult who has lost sight.

It is helpful when parents think of a future for the child to see or be well acquainted with successful blind people in a variety of settings. This might be accomplished by finding successful role models or reading biographies of individuals who have grown up without sight. One example is Robert Russell who became a successful professor of English. And again, this concept applies to adults who become blind or lose sight.

When connecting parents and families with "mentors" professionals should use caution to assure that the blind adult is successful in his/her social and employment life and not assume that just because the person is blind, he or she is typical or has a positive self-concept. Some adults who are blind have gained their current self-concept almost exclusively from social/political groups who wish to perpetuate their particular philosophy and promote one view of how those who are blind are viewed by society and one method for creating a self-concept in the individual. As mentioned earlier, the only characteristic shared by blind people is blindness. It is unlikely that one way of developing a positive self-concept will work for everyone.

Like other challenges, professionals who work with those who have lost their sight as adults must draw on models from work with the sighted to help know what will be helpful for their adult clients. As other chapters have pointed out, personal beliefs and attitudes of the professional will influence what and how services are provided. This is true in helping adults who become blind maintain a healthy self-concept or develop a new one, as discussed by Cholden.

Often in the early stages of rehabilitation, the client focuses on the physical aspects of what he or she can no longer do. The impact of physical limitations is exaggerated relative to the other parts of the self, such as attractiveness, competence, and relationships. The self-concept is damaged by the client's belief that he or she is no longer desirable physically to others, that he or she can no longer be an effective worker, and/or that he or she cannot be a "good" parent, spouse, or friend. Given these doubts, it is important for the rehabilitation program to provide experiences that dispel the negative self-depreciating beliefs.

Children and adults need both formal and informal experience to help teach adaptive skills needed for competence in all aspects of their life. Both successful and unsuccessful experiences, mostly informal, will be needed to help the individual acquire an accurate self-concept. Without a comparison of success and failure, attributes cannot be determined. Interactions with people and with the environment supply the feedback necessary to the development of any self-concept. Successes will build a more positive one and failures a more negative one.

DISCUSSION

As professionals attempt to apply self-concept theory to the visually impaired, and especially as they attempt to measure self concepts, they will find many weaknesses and limitations. Yet, they should recognize that there is value in the concept and its relationship to other rehabilitative and educational factors.

As it has been noted before, professionals must expand their assumptions so aspects of life such as volition, purpose, and persistence can become integral parts of the psychology for human beings. As professionals attempt to apply research findings to their work with children and adults, they find that they (children, students, and clients) do not fit into programs based on much of the current research and that there is far more involved than the overly-simplified notions of behavioristic psychology.

SUGGESTED READINGS

1. Bauman, M. K., & Yoder, N. M. (1966). *Adjustment to blindness reviewed.* Springfield, IL: Charles C Thomas.
2. Russell, R.W. (1992). *To catch an angel: Adventures in a world I cannot see.* Vanguard Press.

Chapter 13

VISION AND MEMORY

INTRODUCTION

An area of psychology which has generated a great deal of research is that of memory. The ability to profit from experience and to successfully interact with the environment are dependent upon retaining in some form of memory a record of those experiences. When one gets older and memory begins to fail, the coping abilities diminish proportionately.

The term "memory" comes from the name of the Greek goddess of memory, Mnemosyne. Interestingly enough, according to Greek mythology, she was also the mother of the Muses, the "patron saints" of the arts and sciences, with Zeus, the head of the gods, as their father. The Greeks seemed to understand that all human artistic and scientific endeavors are dependent upon memory for their success. The term "Mnemosyne" provides the words mnemonics, memory, remember, memorial, etc. "Muse" fosters such words as music, museum, amusement, to muse, and so on.

Researchers have learned that memory has several different facets, each with its own special characteristics and processes. Among these are immediate, short-term, and long-term memory. The processes include selecting, organizing, storing, and retrieving the information received. Loss of memory is referred to as amnesia and refers to either temporary or permanent inability to remember names, places, language, or events.

This chapter will explore some of the research related to memory, then consider vision loss and its influence on memory processes. It will be noted that most psychological, rehabilitative, and educational processes depend on memory as well as forgetting for their success.

OBJECTIVES

At the conclusion of this chapter the reader will be able to:

1. Describe in clear terms the characteristics of immediate, short-term, and long-term memory.
2. Demonstrate understanding of the foundational role of memory in almost all other psychological, rehabilitative, and educational activities.
3. Relate knowledge of memory processes to knowledge of vision loss.
4. Utilize "mnemonic" systems which can be used by children in general, and the visually-impaired in particular, in learning and storing important kinds of knowledge.

Immediate Memory
The Magic of 7 – Plus or Minus 2

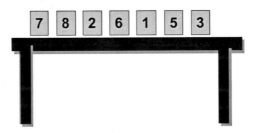

Figure 13.1. Immediate memory begins with sensory information stored in the "sensory register." The sensory register is limited to about seven units of information.

IMMEDIATE MEMORY

Immediate memory is sometimes called the "sensory register." When new materials are presented, the person stores it on a very temporary basis in this memory or sensory register. The amount of information which can be stored in this register is very limited, between five and nine items on average. George Miller described this limitation in a now-famous article entitled, "The Magical Number Seven, Plus or Minus Two." An analogy which helps us understand this register is the placing of items on a desk one at a time, moving each over one position as new items are added, and then dropping the first items off the edge of the desk as more items are added.

Immediate Memory
The Magic of 7 – Plus or Minus 2

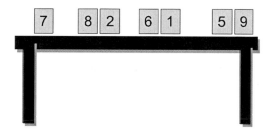

Figure 13.2. Combining small bits of information into single larger units allows more information into the sensory register.

Miller suggested that the learner can circumvent the limited number of "positions" in the register by grouping or lumping items. For example, each position may hold only one coin, but it makes no difference whether the coins are pennies or silver dollars. Thus, the student remembers numbers by "chunking" them as in remembering the prefix of a phone number as a unit rather than as three separate numbers. The projection area for each sensory modality stores information from a specific sense. For example, if you look up a phone number in the book, you will store that number as a visual memory. If you speak the number as you read it, the storage may be in the form of auditory information, or, one could look up the number in a Braille list and remember it as a tactile unit.

Immediate Memory

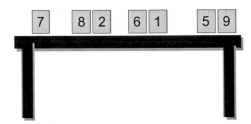

Figure 13.3. Grouping of numbers in telephone directories is an example of "chunking" to make better use of immediate memory.

When the number is retrieved from the memory register, it is best remembered in terms of the sensory modality through which it was input. For many people, it appears to be easier to code the information in several modalities which seems to provide a certain amount of redundancy in retrieval. For education and rehabilitation purposes, the more redundancy, i.e., the more sensory modalities used, the more likely it will be that items can be remembered. The information is stored and retrieved in exactly the form in which it was stored, i.e., the information is not reduced, transformed, or otherwise altered in the process—there is a one-to-one correspondence between input and output.

SHORT-TERM MEMORY

Information stored in the sensory register may or may not be transferred to short-term memory. If it is transferred, it is transferred in terms of the sensory modality used in input and output, but it is also transformed as an "abstract" of the original information.

Taking liberties with the desk analogy, one might think of items that fall may fall into a small basket. Some items will land in the basket, while others fall directly to the floor and become lost. The items in the basket may be inspected to determine how important they are and how useful they may become to learning and actions.

Short-Term Memory

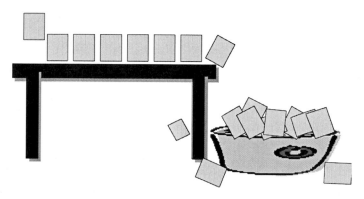

Figure 13.4. When more information transfers from immediate memory to short-term memory, some information is lost.

During the period of time information is stored in short-term memory, it is reduced in volume and detail. Approximately 90 percent is lost over the roughly 24-hour period of short-term memory. Readers have probably seen the "forgetting curve" in a psychology textbook. The information in short-term memory is condensed or abstracted so one can remember the content, but in one's own words or images. Shortly after one listens to a lecture, he/she will probably not be able to remember many of the exact words used to convey an idea, but he/she will recall the idea, or, he/she may condense several ideas into a more general idea. Short-term memory is very fragile, i.e., emotional or physical trauma may interfere with storage of information. Storage is also affected by interfering experiences. This suggests that storage space in short-term memory may be limited, though it is still far greater than in immediate memory.

LONG-TERM MEMORY

Perhaps carrying our analogy too far, one could think of taking the basket of items which were selected for possible use and sorting them according to their most important uses and then cross-referencing

Long-Term Memory

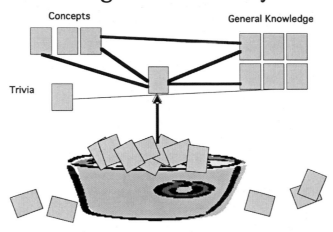

Figure 13.5. More information is lost when transferred to long-term memory but, when stored, is more stable as it is integrated into concepts and relationships from a variety of sensory perception sources.

them to other possible categories and uses. The items would be in a storage medium that would last indefinitely, but use of an item would automatically bring up the cross-references for inspection and possible use.

Unlike immediate memory and short-term memory, long-term memory has information coded in several sensory modalities, has unlimited storage capacity, is very robust or resistant to loss, and is retrieved through use of many different strategies. When information is transferred from short-term to long-term memory, many aspects of the information are used to code for storage. For example, one might note the sound of the name of a person, the way it looks in written form, words with which it rhymes, the facial characteristics of the person whose name it is, and many other things one might know about that person, etc. One may be able to retrieve the name from storage by using any of the information "pegs" with which it was associated such as gender, location of residence, rhyming sounds, occupation, etc.

Wilder Penfield, a world-renowned neurologist at the Montreal Neurological Institute, has conducted research which strongly suggests that everything to which people have attended is stored in the tissues of the brain. Evidence from hypnosis also supports this idea. This would suggest that storage is not the problem in memory loss but, rather, the ability to retrieve the information. It may well be that the associations between what is stored and other stored information may not be strong or may be difficult to retrieve also.

Coding of information in long-term memory does not appear to be in specific brain "addresses," but rather is spread throughout the brain. This would support the finding that memory is stored in many different ways through associations with concepts or categories. All of the connections may not be retrievable from any one part of the brain, but enough would be available to recall something about the information which is meaningful. Karl Pribram from Stanford University has suggested that memory is stored like an "hologram" in which each small piece of the original picture contains enough of the total information to retrieve the essential picture.

Information is stored in long-term memory without thought or action on an individual's part. However, if one does take specific actions to establish meaningful associations between new and old information, it is possible to retrieve what is wanted purposefully much better. A number of "mnemonic devices" or memory aids have been developed which have been shown to assist in information retrieval. Among these are:

1. Poems or rhymes such as commercials or "Thirty days hath September, April, June and November; 31 hath all the rest, save February which alone has 28."
2. Peg-words which can be associated with the new information to form mental images. When the peg-word is recalled, the new information associated with it is also retrieved. The peg words are memorized in a framework so they can be associated with the information which is to be stored and retrieved, i.e., the first sound of words in an easily remembered sentence match a list of items that begin with the same sound. For example, "Mrs. Vanheppleberg eats marshmallows just sitting under new porches" could be matched with the order of planets from the sun Mercury, Venus, Earth, Mars, Jupiter, Saturn, Uranus, Neptune, and Pluto.
3. Number-to-letter conversions which allow numbers to be translated into consonants which, in turn can be combined with vowels to form words. For example, you might associate 2 with "H,"

3 with "D," and 7 with "R." If you saw the 473, you would transform the digits to HRD which can be made into the word "herd" or "hard" by the addition of a vowel which carries no information. You could use the new word to form an image which would facilitate recall of the number.

4. Word-associations such as bread-butter, cold-hot, or mountain-clouds. If you were given one of the words in the pair, you would recall the word not given.

5. The Method of Loci, in which you select a specific location such as a room, a house, or a block. You would identify, in advance, a set of characteristics or locations within the unit such as pieces of furniture in a room which would then be used to form mental images with the new materials to be stored and retrieved.

These and other memory aids can be used to learn items or elements in a series such as a shopping list or elements in an assignment or often-needed information such as addresses or famous quotations. Some small children have difficulty in learning the days of the week, the names of the states, or a sequence of computer instructions. It should be possible in some instances to devise a memory aid which they can use in making it easier to recall at an appropriate time.

VISION LOSS AND MEMORY

Research has shown that visually-impaired children, on average, score higher on short-term memory tasks than do sighted children. But because it is more difficult for visually-impaired children to use some memory aids typically used by the sighted such as paper and pencil, notebooks, and lists of phone numbers posted on the wall, they learn to rely more heavily on memory. This is a plausible explanation for the improved performance on memory tasks. It does not, however, support the idea that nature has compensated a person with vision loss by providing an improved memory.

On the other hand, visually-impaired children appear to have fewer concepts derived from the world of experience. This would seemingly limit their use of preexisting concepts as memory aids for storing and retrieving new information. An alert teacher can assist a person to develop clearly-defined concepts and then teach how these concepts can be used to assist memory processes.

DISCUSSION

In the not-too-distant past people relied far more on oral transmission of culture than on the printed page. Some societies even had specific individuals who were given the responsibility of memorizing all about some period of history and then reproducing those memories upon demand for the benefit of others. Japan provides an example of this. They had individuals who worked as an apprentice with a master who was responsible for knowing all the historical information about a particular dynasty. In most instances, the "repository" individuals were blind and this occupation was reserved for blind children.

People now live in an information age. It is impossible for them to store in their minds all the information available and which they need. Rather than memorizing the actual information, people typically learn only where and how the information is stored. Educators and rehabilitation workers need to know how to access this information and they need to teach their clients and students how to do so. This is a particular problem, however, for the visually impaired. Braille, large-type books, recordings, etc. are far too limited in quantity and quality to keep up with the need. Perhaps computers will help, but they are not the total answer. Maybe they need to call on their clients to improve their memory functions so they can better organize and take responsibility for information searches. Perhaps they can improve both human and mechanical information storage by understanding better how their memories work and how memory processes can be enhanced.

SUGGESTED READINGS

1. Miller, G. (1956). The magical number seven, plus or minus two: Some limits on our capacity for processing information. *Psychological Review, 63*, 81–97.

2. Penfield, W. *Speech and brain mechanisms.* Princeton, NY: Princeton University Press.

3. Pribram, C. (1971). *Language of the brain: Experimental paradoxes in neural psychology.* New York: Prentice-Hall.

Chapter 14

ORIENTATION AND MOBILITY

INTRODUCTION

Among the major problems associated with vision loss is the ability to move about freely in and around the environment and to interact with it. Few problems pose greater challenges to the person with a vision loss than getting where he or she wants to go when one wants to go. This problem is referred to under the general term "orientation and mobility–O&M." For those new to work with individuals who are blind or who have severe low vision, these two aspects of independent travel need to be defined and analyzed.

Orientation has been defined as "knowledge of where one is in relation to other parts of the environment." As an example, if you want to go to the post office, you must, first of all, know where you are at the moment, where the post office is in relation to where you are, and how to move so as to arrive there.

Mobility is "the ability to move from one place to another and to avoid dangers or obstacles along the way." This movement can be actually moving yourself, as by walking, or traveling on a vehicle. Rivers, mountains, oceans, fences, walls, utility poles, etc. constitute some of the obstacles to be avoided.

For the visually impaired, these concepts have special importance since both must be performed with little or no assistance from eyesight, and this is complicated in many cases by lack of knowledge of the world in general.

Techniques and devices have been developed to assist the person with vision loss to become an independent traveler, but, even with these aids, only a relatively small percentage of persons with visual impairments have achieved a significant level of independence. This is partly due to the fact that more than half of the population of visually impaired are elderly and have additional motor or sensory problems. Also, a significant number of children have additional motor and intellectual disabilities.

This chapter will consider in detail some of the physical and psychological aspects of independent travel. It will also consider the role of the special teacher, the regular classroom teacher, rehabilitation worker, family, and others in the development of good travel skills. Last, the chapter will consider ways in which independent travel can be improved for children and adults with visual impairments.

OBJECTIVES

At the completion of this chapter the reader will be able to:

1. Define and discuss the concepts "orientation," "mobility," "independent traveler," "spatial awareness," etc. and how these relate to children or adults with vision loss.
2. Identify nonvisual information which can be used to accomplish personal independent travel for individual children and adults necessary for meaningful O&M.
3. Recognize and modify aspects of the environment which constitute hazards and barriers to the person with vision loss so that independent travel is more likely to occur.

MOBILITY

Think about the means by which human beings and animals achieve movement, i.e., the means by which they move from one place to another. These, of course, include walking, running, jumping, hopping, skipping, flying, driving, swimming, leaping and leapfrogging, rolling, somersaulting, shuffling, waddling, etc., etc. Depending on the physical characteristics of the individual traveler and the environment in which the organism exists, some of these means are more appropriate than others for getting about. Some of these movement techniques are developed through maturation and learning, and move from simple to more complex modes. The young bird is nest bound until it matures to the point that it can fly, first with difficulty to virtual effortless flight. The human infant crawls, creeps, scoots, walks, runs, skips, strolls, jogs, rides a tricycle, rides a bicycle, and eventually learns to drive a car—and then loses all of these earlier skills. Boats, ships, helicopters, airplanes, rockets, trains, submarines, etc. have been developed to make humans more mobile.

For most human beings, the use of sight is an essential part of the process of movement. Vision is particularly important in identifying and avoiding obstacles. Vision also provides feedback about progress toward desired, distant goals.

There are other factors which affect movement. One must have the physical qualities associated with specific movements such as strength, dexterity, flexibility, endurance and stamina, balance, coordination, etc. The person who has lost a leg is, of necessity, limited in the ability to run or walk. Damage to the ankles, knees, and hips greatly reduces mobility. The bird must have wings and feathers, together with light, hollow bones, and muscles before flight is possible. If the feathers are cut off or plucked, flight becomes difficult or impossible.

People tend to take their movement abilities for granted unless they become involved in sports requiring special concentration and practice, or until they are hampered in movement. This is certainly true for basic mobility skills. They become aware of individual skills used in complex movements such as walking or running when they are pushed to the limits of present competence.

Most people do not realize what an amazing skill bipedal walking is. They move one leg forward which throws them off balance. They bring the second leg forward to catch themselves, then follow with the first leg again. In reality, legs are like the spokes in a wheel which are brought forward rather than rotating around the hub of the wheel. In the case of humans, the hub is their center of gravity which must be kept as nearly as possible over the end of the spoke: the foot.

For most people, walking is very easy until someone asks exactly how it is done. People are like the centipede which got along fine until it was asked which foot it moved first.

ORIENTATION

Orientation is more difficult to understand than is mobility. It appears to require the development of a mental image or picture of the world, with more specific pictures and maps of the immediate location. The traveler must be able to identify specific landmarks, and then, both mentally and physically, move from that locus by moving in a particular direction. The direction is considered in terms of a direction scheme, usually the right-left directions or the points of a compass.

For example, if one wishes to go to the post office, as mentioned above, he/she must know where he/she is. This is determined by observing landmarks or other signs which they can compare with their mental pictures or maps. If they do not have mental pictures or maps, or if they cannot recognize landmarks, they are "lost." The ability to recognize familiar locations is an extremely complex process which is not well understood, though attempts to create robots which can even remotely duplicate this ability has not met with much success. To a large extent, the recognition of landmarks is based on visual perception, though people can use hearing as well when they hear traffic noise or the sound of a waterfall to identify their whereabouts.

Next, they must know where their desired destination—the post office—is located. This may be an actual mental image, or an address in a context with which they are familiar. In other words, they will need to know when they have reached their goal. The difficulty in recognizing their goal is also complex. If one has never been to the address before, many mental elements are necessary to determine if the current location fits criteria needed in a particular situation to reach the desired destination.

Third, people need to know something about a route which will take them from where they are to where they want to go. They can turn to the right or to the left or go straight ahead, proceed a certain distance, then turn in a specific direction, etc., etc. The turn points involve identifiable landmarks also, e.g., a street sign, a building of a given description, a given number of blocks, etc. A specific map with identified turn or choice points gives a specific route which may or may not be the most efficient, direct, or simplest route. It may also suffer from confusion as to the specific landmarks which are to be used in the identification of choice points.

An alternative method for moving from Point A to Point B is the use of a compass, either an actual physical instrument or an internalized mental compass. In this method of orientation, the individual must have a "big picture" of the two locations and their relation to one another. This approach allows considerable flexibility in choice of a route because it is not necessary to know specific landmarks in order to make decisions at choice points. So long as one is moving in the general direction of the destination, many alternative routes are possible. For example, if one wanted to get from San Antonio, Texas to Austin, Texas he/she could take any number of streets which open toward the north. One can choose the street which seems to offer the fewest obstacles in the form of stops or traffic.

One factor in independent travel often overlooked by students of these phenomena is that of purpose or intent of travel. One does not go to a place for no reason at all. There is usually a motivational component involved. The motivational components involves factors such as one's needs, wants and attitudes toward his/her ability to get to the destination, awareness of potential obstacles or problems in the move, the strength of the desire to move out, and the perseverance in pursuing the goal. Any or all of these factors can influence the choice of movement and its direction. As an example, what explains why some people climb mountains? Unless one knows what the motive for that action is, it would not be easily explained, what with the dangers and difficulties involved. Climbers explain their "mad" behaviors with a number of different reasons ranging from the challenge of the task to the desire to see what one can observe from the summit. Without an intent which benefits the traveler, it is unlikely that significant effort will be made to travel to any destination.

When one does not have or loses eyesight, all three of these factors are altered. Most of the activities which motivate sighted individuals to develop physical skills are not important for the blind. Many of these activities involve some danger or difficulty for individuals without sight. Hence, many individuals with visual handicaps are not in very "good physical shape." Their muscles are flaccid, their aerobic potential is greatly limited, they have very little physical endurance, and their coordination is poor from lack of practice in using the skills involved in travel. As a consequence, many visually-impaired children and adults cannot travel with ease or efficiency.

Though adults who lose their sight developed the skills necessary for independent travel from childhood, their fears often lead them to settle into a sedentary life. Lack of activity soon leads to many of the same physical problems as children without sight have. Without continued physical and social activities, many of their former interests also wane. Physical conditioning is essential if children and adults who are blind are to be effective and efficient travelers.

Orientation in space, as noted above, relies on visual cues. For example, most buildings do not produce recognizable auditory or tactual signals which can be used to identify them. Sidewalks, curbs, gutters, flaws in the pavement, grass, etc. can be used as substitutes for visual cues, but these are not nearly as accessible as are visual perceptions nor as clear-cut.

New systems located on buildings and landmarks within buildings that transmit signals to receivers used by persons who are blind are being tested and installed to make identification possible. Similar devices are placed on public transit vehicles. This is not a widespread aid in most buildings or cities but has potential for making independent travel easier for those who are blind. Global positioning devices with speech components also hold promise for identification of a person's present location.

Spatial awareness, knowing what environmental aspects fill the space around one, is also limited for the person without or with limited sight. The size, shape, contours, and textures of buildings are almost entirely lacking as useful cues for identification. Mountains or tall buildings as landmarks may be far less obvious or meaningful to the traveler. In other words, the visual elements of the environment which are so readily available to the sighted must have substitute cues. These may be of less help to the traveler. Street signs, room numbers, doorways, stairs, etc. are of no practical use to one who cannot access them in some way other than sight. Since the implementation of the Americans with Disabilities Act (ADA), Progress has been made in providing accessible signage in public building. However, locating the signs themselves can be a difficult task for some blind persons.

Even more difficult than finding sensory identification cues is the development of a mental map by the person without sight. Sight, in contrast to touch, hearing, or kinesthesia, is capable of providing a Gestalt or overall form of the environment quickly and efficiently. Many elements can be experienced concurrently with sight. For persons who are blind, other senses provide sequential information which must be held in memory while elements are experienced and finally put together to form the whole. The more complex the object or environment to be experienced, the greater the cognitive strain involved in developing the mental image or map. Even with superior short-term memory, the task is formidable if a useful map is to be created. Models or tactile maps may help, but the scale to be used in relating the model to the real world is, in itself, difficult to understand without visual experience. If you have never seen an elephant except as a small model, how can you understand just how large a real elephant is?

Motivations for travel by children and adults with visual impairments do not differ from those of the sighted except that mobility for one without sight involves a much greater sense of danger and difficulty than it does for one with sight. The intense mental alertness needed to travel safely and the training in use of any mobility aides takes considerable effort. In short, a person without sight will usually need a stronger incentive to travel than a person with sight. This, in turn, makes it more likely that the person with a visual impairment will not obtain adequate exercise, hence making it more difficult to be in good shape for travel purposes.

Another factor related to travel for the blind is the relatively high rate of unemployment among the visually disabled. Whether lack of travel ability inhibits employment, or whether the lack of employment inhibits the tendency to travel is a question needing further research. It seems clear, however, that a person who cannot travel to and from a place of employment is not likely to be employed.

Age is another factor. Readers will recall that about half of the legally blind are above the age of 65. Not only do people in this age group experience more physical problems which interfere with independent travel, they also often lack many of the incentives which influence younger people to travel. The direction of cause-and-effect relationships are not clear here, but there is a general tendency for older people to slow down and seek activities which do not require extensive mobility

THE SIXTH SENSE

Readers have probably heard about the so-called "sixth sense" of the blind. From earliest times, some blind people have been able to detect the presence of an obstacle in one's path. The sensation has been described as a feeling of warmth or pressure on the forehead and cheeks. The closer one approaches the obstacle, the stronger the sensations.

About 50 years ago, a group of researchers at Cornell University decided to investigate this phenomenon and did so with remarkable success. In fact, many psychology texts hold this research up as an excellent example of quality research.

To summarize what they found in a very brief manner, they found that this so-called "facial vision" is, in fact, related to high-frequency—above 10,000 Hertz—sound waves which are not "heard" but "felt." It is, to some extent, like the echo-location ability of bats and porpoises.

The subjects used in these studies included both blind and blindfolded children. It was found that, after a few days during which the sighted subjects were taught what to attend to, there was no difference in the ability of the subjects to use facial vision. Later studies found that, with training, some subjects can identify shapes by the sound patterns reflected from the surfaces of the shapes.

Riley, Luterman, and Cohen, in a study of the relationship between high-frequency hearing ability and mobility, found a strong, negative relationship between hearing loss and mobility skill. Unfortunately, high-frequency hearing ability information is not readily available for evaluating blind people's potential as independent travelers. Further, this finding is significant for older individuals since with presbycupia there is a loss of high frequency hearing incident to aging.

Cratty has identified another ability through research on blind subjects which has meaning for mobility. This is a "veering tendency." When walking without sight as a guide, a person will have a tendency to veer to the right or left in a consistent manner. The amount of veer will vary for different children and adults, but it can be determined and skill in correcting veer will help minimize its impact on travel. A localized sound source can also be used as a beacon which can play the same role as a visual cue in keeping one on track. In the natural environment, there are few such sound beacons.

MOBILITY AIDS

Several fairly effective mobility aids have been developed to assist the visually impaired travel more effectively. All of these aids have limitations, however, which means that researchers still need to continue work on developing new and better approaches. One of the more recent innovations is the use of robotic vehicles that can lead or be programmed to support mobility. Some of the more common mobility aids are discussed next.

1. ***Sighted Guide.*** The assistance of a person with sight as a guide for a person with vision loss is an ancient method for getting about. This approach helps resolve both obstacle avoidance and orientation problems. The sighted guide can use an easily-learned technique in which the blind person can know by the actions of the guide when turns are to be made, when there are intersections, when to go both up and down steps or curbs, when the passageway is narrow, and when to start or stop. This is all done without the necessity of speech so conversation can continue for other communication needs. The major limitation with this method of travel assistance is that it requires two people to go where only one needs or wants to go. It is, therefore, inefficient. It also fosters greater dependence rather than creating personal responsibility. It can also be awkward when two people are going in tight quarters. The method, nonetheless, is a very useful and necessary one for some people at particular times and in specific locations. Each person working with the visually impaired needs to develop proficiency in use of "sighted guide" techniques and practices.

2. ***Dog Guide.*** There are records of blind people being led by dogs which go far back into history. The first systematic approach to the use of dog guides for the blind occurred in Germany during and after World War I. German Shepherd dogs, noted for their intelligence and strong devotion to a master were trained to identify and avoid obstacles in the path of the blind master.

Wide use of dog guides was later brought to the United State when the Seeing Eye was established. Since the first school was launched in the 1920s other training schools have been established. Education and rehabilitation agencies maintain or have access to dog guide training program throughout the country.

It is generally not recognized that dogs are mobility aids almost exclusively. They are not orientation aids. Dogs allow a blind person to travel with a great deal of confidence and with relative safety so long as the master can give directions to the dog. Using a dog guide allows the persons who is blind to use public transportation and have access to almost all public places.

There is often a misconception that the dog guide can merely be told things like take me to the store, work, etc. It may be true that through routines a dog appears to "know" everything about travel. In fact, the major drawback is that dogs do not have a cognitive map which would allow them to be told where the blind person wishes to go. The blind person must have the mental map and be responsible for the orientation aspects of travel. Another drawback is that dogs need to be cared for—fed, groomed, toilette, etc. and they grow ill and old. It is also expensive to train both the dog and the blind traveler, though many schools or philanthropic organizations pay these costs.

3. *The Long Cane.* From earliest times, some blind people have been able to get about with the assistance of a staff or short cane which was used by the sighted for support, but by the blind as a probe. The method was unsystematic and ineffective in strange areas because these staffs and short canes were not designed to detect obstacles.

After World War II, Dr. Richard Hoover, under assignment from the Department of Defense, developed the use of the "long cane." This cane, unlike the short cane, was not used for support, but as a tactile probe used as a means to identify a clear path in front of the traveler. The cane tests the surface upon which the next step will fall, and gives information about the texture of the surface. The cane is swung in rhythm with the footsteps from side to side so it touches the surface where the next step would occur. This technique, in familiar areas and with a good "shore line" to follow allows rapid walking with good safety. The cane detects drop-offs, but does not detect, obviously, overhead obstructions such as tree limbs and guy wires.

Extensive training is required for the development of travel proficiency with the long cane, but the cane is relatively inexpensive. It requires virtually no care, and is ready to go where and when the traveler is.

4. *Electronic Aids.* A number of electronic guidance devices have been developed, some of which incorporate the cane with a sonar-like feedback from the environment. An example of this is the "laser cane" which has three laser sensors which monitor for obstacles at head level, directly in front of the traveler, and drop-offs. The cane itself also helps in detecting obstacles, especially drop offs. It has limitations because of the electronic components. This device is also expensive.

Another electronic aid is the "Sonic Guide" which also uses sound waves to provide feedback from the environment. This particular device was developed by Dr. Leslie Kay, an electrical engineer from The University of Canterbury in Christchurch, New Zealand. There are several versions of this device, but the most common is a head-held device which emits a cone-shaped ultrasound signal in front of the traveler. This ultrasound is reflected back to transducers which send a sound signal to each ear, giving a stereophonic signal. One can determine the location of obstacles, their surface texture, and distance by differences in the frequency of the pitch and quality of signals. The hands remain free to hold a cane for identifying surface characteristics and drop offs or for carrying handbags or other materials.

The major drawbacks of this device are high costs and extensive training use requires. Like the laser cane, some information concerning overhead obstacles is provided, but wires or small branches might not be detected.

These electronic devices are mobility aids, not orientation aids. Some attempts have been made to provide an electronic signal which could be used as a distance reference point to aid navigation, but these are too expensive for installation in every part of the environment, and do not allow the user much flexibility in choice of route. Some groups of the blind have objected to their installation since they tend to be too specifically tied to a route and the information does not provide assistance away from the "area of coverage" of the system.

ACQUIRING INDEPENDENT TRAVEL

People with visual impairments, like their sighted peers, develop independent travel skills over a long period of time. One would not expect that a young child would be able to travel in a city environment without adult supervision. By the same token, the person with a vision loss must gradually acquire independent travel skills which will start from specific, safe environments to more and more remote and less well-known areas. The home environment is mastered before the person can move out into the neighborhood and the areas beyond. This expanding world of the person will require, for the visually-impaired person, greater utilization of travel aids when necessary and appropriate. Some mobility specialists advocate the use of miniaturized canes for very young blind children for travel assistance in a limited environment. This would avoid some tendencies for blind children to acquire poor habits of posture and gait, while providing safety and encouragement in moving about the limited environment which in turn would encourage development of strength, coordination, stamina, posture, and gait. Other mobility specialists fear that blind children would be encouraged by too early use of the cane to extend their travel beyond the bounds of safety. The issue is still open.

The ultimate goal of mobility training for the blind person is the ability to travel safely and independently in an efficient, effective, and graceful manner in both familiar and unfamiliar environments. It would seem that even very young infants need some motivation to overcome the inertia inhibiting movement, and this would be especially true for children with a vision loss. As a matter of fact, Hart has observed significant differences between blind and sighted infants in their acceptance of the prone position, a necessary posturing needed for crawling and creeping. The difference seems to derive from the lack of interesting visual stimuli which would attract the attention of the blind child. As the normal child grows older, imitation becomes a strong incentive to walk, run, jump, etc., but the child with a vision loss often lacks awareness of the mobility model being provided. Still later, this lack of a model and motivation to move impedes progress toward independent travel. If this is to be remedied, some substitute incentives and models must be provided if the goals of O&M are to be realized.

The above-mentioned problems do not exhaust the list of possible inhibitors to mobility on the part of children and adults with vision loss, but they are examples of the kinds of elements which need to be included in an individual plan for orientation and mobility training. All the factors listed earlier, including such things as strength, flexibility, stamina, coordination, etc. need to be included, where appropriate, in the plan for achieving independent travel.

Another group of concepts which should be used in developing elements in a travel training program are recognition of nonvisual cues which can, perhaps, be used as cues or landmarks by the person with the vision loss. For example, the odor coming from a barber shop, a grocery store, service station, tire store, bake shop, or flower vendor can be used to identify one's present location. Sounds made by exhaust fans, street traffic, water fountains, air conditioners, etc. can also be used as landmarks.

Characteristics of the walking surface can also yield identifiable cues for location such as grass, cement, asphalt, up and down grades, oil slicks, puddles, curbs, etc. The alert teacher can explore an environment, be alert for these elements, and be conscious of ways by which a person without vision could be taught what these cues are and how they can be used in mobility. It will undoubtedly take many, many months or years of efforts in this area before children and adults are able to form mental images and maps. The ability to construct concepts for mobility and concept acquisition must not be left to chance. Adults will have trouble adjusting to the loss of sight but will have the advantage of visual memory to form their mental maps and concepts. However, use of nonvisual cues should not be left to chance for them and specific instruction should be a part of their training program.

DISCUSSION

The ideas summarized in this chapter are only some of the areas which make up entire graduate programs and, therefore, the reader should consider this chapter as introductory. He/she will recognize, however, that many parts of the mobility training of visually-impaired children and adults are things which the teachers and others who are not orientation and mobility specialists can work on in preparation for more detailed and concentrated efforts of mobility specialists. Such factors as general physical fitness and cognitive development are not limited to mobility but need to be developed for their own sake.

It should also be recognized that most sighted, nonspecialists in vision, such as educators in the public schools and employers will have little or no awareness of the factors which make independent travel for the visually impaired possible. It is, therefore, imperative that a vision specialist be willing to be firm in insisting that mobility be included in any education, rehabilitation, or placement plan. It may well be true that many families, for a variety of reasons, may not be aware of the importance of independent travel as a major goal of the education of the visually impaired. However, vocational choices, place of residence, leisure-time activities, and even marriage possibilities will be greatly influenced by the presence of graceful and effective mobility. Mobility skills will NOT develop automatically; they must be planned for and incorporated into the curriculum for children and adults with visual handicaps.

SUGGESTED READINGS

1. Cratty, B.J. (1967). The Perception of gradient and the veering tendency while walking without vision. *Research Bulletin,* American Foundation for the Blind, *14,* 31–51.
2. Luterman, D.M., Melrose, J., Welsh, R.L. (1963). Auditory response in selected elderly men. *Journal of Gerontology, 18,* 267–280.
3. Welsh, R.L., & Blasch, B.B. (eds.). *Foundations of orientation and mobility.* New York: American Foundation for the Blind.

Chapter 15

ADVOCACY

INTRODUCTION

The last 50 years have seen a highly significant shift in the most prevalent place for education of children with visual impairments–from the residential school to the local public school. This shift has not been an unmixed blessing. The reading and writing of Braille have diminished; independent travel has become more difficult; the transition from school to advanced training and employment is more diverse and inconsistent, with rural students often being forced to move to urban areas or to be left without services; public attitudes toward children without sight and with visual disability have not improved; and the favorable legislative provisions for services for the visually impaired have been diluted as other vocal minorities have demanded special consideration. The roles of professionals working with the visually impaired have also changed remarkably during this same time period. Generally, these highly trained professionals provide less direct service to meet the specific needs of the visually impaired than decades ago.

This chapter will focus on one aspect of the changing role of such professionals, viz., advocacy. Parent groups, families, and organizations of and for the blind must team with individual workers and professional organizations to ensure that children and adults with visual impairments receive the kinds of services which will allow them to become fully functional and contributing members of society, to become tax payers rather than tax consumers, and to experience meaningful and rewarding lives. Individuals with visual impairments as well as education, rehabilitation, and social service systems must cooperate to ensure that those who are blind or have low vision receive services they are entitled to and that they are appropriate and meet quality standards.

The direct service provider should be a primary interface and conduit for information and support to those who are blind or have low vision. To fulfil the role, he or she must first have the desire and commitment to place the needs of each client as his/her highest priority. Next, he or she must develop the knowledge of what children and adults with visual impairments need in general and in particular what they must do to be able to succeed in life. Then, he or she must develop skills necessary to work with families, colleagues, and administrators in order to develop an appropriate individualized educational and/or rehabilitation plan for each person. And finally, he or she must work to ensure that the resources are available and used wisely to carry out the plan, including his/her own services.

OBJECTIVES

Upon completion of this chapter readers will be able to:

1. Identify a procedure to be used in the development of an individualized plan for a particular person with visual impairments.
2. Recognize sources of potential difficulties in bringing all concerned to a mutually-agreed upon plan for children or adults with visual impairments.
3. Identify resources at the local, state, and national levels and develop a plan for tapping those resources in order to implement education and/or rehabilitation programs.

FAMILIES AS PARTNERS

In the past, parents were the forgotten or silent "partners" in the education of exceptional children. PL 94–142 (All Handicapped Children's Education Act of 1975) later named the Individuals with Disabilities Education Act (IDEA), however, mandates that parents be an integral part of the education program planning process.

Nevertheless, because having a child who is blind or has low vision is not a common experience, many parents do not know what their child needs, how their child's program is to be developed, and in which ways they should become involved. Parents and families can and should be one of the most valuable supports in doing the job of providing appropriate services. Too often, parents are believed to be less knowledgeable and competent and expected to accept without question what professionals in their child's life tell them. This attitude should be avoided. Even if parents did not have information to share about their child, which they most certainly do, professionals must take the responsibility of informing them about their rights and responsibilities.

Professionals can work closely with parents in identifying the long-term goals for the child who is blind or has low vision, the resources necessary to reach those goals, and the activities necessary for the child's plan implementation. Professionals and the parents must be in agreement on these elements *before* the IEP meeting. Although other team members should be consulted before, during, and after planning meetings, parents are the key to success as a teacher and as the recognized "expert" for meeting individual needs of the child. For example, teachers and the parents may realize that mobility training will be essential for a person's future entry into the labor force. Other professionals may not understand this and will attempt to have such training delayed or omitted from the current education plan on grounds that the district cannot afford such services or cannot obtain the services of a qualified mobility specialist. But, if the professional in work for the visually impaired and the parents agree upon the need and work together, they will be successful in having orientation and mobility services included in the education program.

In a like manner, families of adult rehabilitation clients must be involved in the development of an individualized rehabilitation plan, and the family could provide similar kinds of assistance as do the parents of a visually impaired child in school situations. One difference in the rehabilitation planning process is that client choice becomes the driving force. This difference is significant. Case workers must provide information so the person who is blind can make an informed decision about the services he or she will receive. The process also places responsibility on the client to follow through on the agreed upon plan for rehabilitation services.

THE INDIVIDUAL PLAN

In a simplified form, the process for developing an individual plan for education or for rehabilitation consists of the following steps:

First, the person must be identified as having a visual disability. This may include providing evidence of meeting specific criteria such as legal blindness or specific visual acuities in order to qualify for services.

Second is an assessment of the needs the person has that are caused by the lack of sight. This is often viewed as a discrepancy between what is expected or desired and where the present level of functioning is. It is sometime helpful to develop a list of the skills required to overcome the difference between present functioning levels and future goals.

Third is selection of services that meet the needs identified during the assessment. This should include: (a) the type of professional who will do the training or provide the service, (b) the amount of time training or services will be provided, (c) any adaptations to the training program, (d) special aids or equipment, (e) alternative materials and media, (f) adaptive technology, (g) other support services needed during training such as transportation and therapy, and (h) goals for future placements. Fourth is a description of the setting in which the training and services will be provided. For children, services may be through a residential school, resource room in a public school, itinerant teaching services, or consultation with regular classroom teachers or others. Adult training could be in a training/adjustment center, a technical school, a college or university, or within the person's home. The key is to describe the appropriate setting to meet individually established goals.

Finally, a time should be set to review progress, do additional assessments if needed, make changes, and establish new goals when necessary. This step is meant to assure that the plan is being carried out and to determine when goals have been met. These steps can be repeated as often as needed in order to progress toward and meet long-term goals.

Perhaps the largest barrier to successful implementation of individual education and rehabilitation plans is the current shortage of trained personnel for the assessment and training of children and adults with visual impairments. This is a situation that needs advocates to petition for funding to support the needed staff and to recruit capable students to enter the field. Due to the shortage of trained personnel, professionals who do exist must attempt to fill this void by being aware of resources for obtaining meaningful assessments and other services and using them to full advantage. In this area of responsibility, workers need to regularly read professional journals, participate in in-service programs, and attend professional meetings on a continuing basis if they are to keep abreast of what is needed and available. The appropriate answer to this dilemma is to have adequate numbers of trained professionals in work for the blind who are trained and able to perform assessments and training needed by students and clients who are blind or have a severe loss of sight.

All professionals should maintain a resource file which includes information about each of the national organizations concerned with the field of vision loss. All of them should be contacted systematically for the latest description of their activities, the best way to contact them, and how to procure their services. Most large agencies have internet websites, 1-800 numbers, or other easily accessible ways to communicate.

In addition to national support agencies and organizations, there are local groups and chapters of national organizations with which professionals should become familiar. Among these are learning resource centers, schools for the blind, rehabilitation services for the visually impaired, library services for the blind, the local affiliate of the American Council of the Blind (ACB), the local affiliate of the National Federation of the Blind (NFB), Prevent Blindness, local Lions Clubs, the Chapter of the Association for Education and Rehabilitation for the Blind and Visually Impaired (AER), and local chapters of the National Association for Parents of the Visually Impaired (NAPVI). A listing of mailing addresses and phone numbers of these local resources will be very useful. Professionals who are not already a member of one or more of these groups, should consider such memberships that both support their activities and ask for their assistance when needed. These groups can be especially helpful in supporting legislative and funding issues.

Through the above-mentioned organizations, the reader will become acquainted with other individuals who work with children and adults with visual disabilities. One will also become acquainted with individuals who have visual impairments themselves. There are still other resources in professional, business, religious, and civic organizations in and around local communities. In addition, government workers and officials learn of and can become strong advocates for individual and program needs. The list of possible supports and sources of advocacy are almost limitless but need a conscious effort to find and encourage them to give support.

Sharing information about what one provides and how the services benefit individuals is the major way to build advocacy. The more professionals try to share with others about the work they are doing and the more "networks" they become a part of, the more effective advocacy efforts will become in meeting the needs of individuals. For example, when a particular person needs a service not available through an agency, professionals or families may have to seek assistance from another agency from outside the field of work for the blind if that service is to become available. For another example, if a person is interested in Amateur Radio both as a hobby and as a potential avenue to a career, he/she may need to contact a local "ham" radio operator or the local amateur radio club or the amateur-radio affiliate of the American Council of the Blind (with which the local group of blind people is affiliated) to get the help they need.

Searching and becoming knowledgeable about all sources of support and advocacy within the community will require teachers, rehabilitation workers, and all who serve the blind to have a professional commitment which goes beyond the usual working hours. And, while professionals must not neglect their own family and have a personal life outside of work, they must consider the children and adults with whom they work as "their" children, friends, and associates.

EFFECTIVE ADVOCACY METHODS

How one advocates for oneself or on behalf of others is important. Though highly personality dependent, there is a "right" way and a "wrong" way to go about helping students or clients to achieve their goals or to improve services. The following are suggestions of how to advocate effectively.

1. Speak up early and at the immediate level. Often a simple conversation which clearly states issues or concerns is the most effective means for getting changes in services. Follow the "chain of command." Going to a program director's, superintendent, department director, legislator, or governor before working at the lower levels of administration seldom has positive results. In most cases, the first question will be, "Have you talked with the teacher, counselor, etc.?" Even if the problem cannot be solved until court proceedings are begun, the courts will expect that all "administrative remedies" have been exhausted. Put things in writing and keep a written log of meetings contacts and other efforts.

2. Distribute well-written memos, letters and brochures. This can be of great help in letting people know the needs of clients and programs. Complaints, requests, and information are often stated best in writing to assure that all who see them have the same information and to document the complaint or request. One thing to remember is that putting things in writing increases the formality of the discussion and may not be as effective as face to face conversations. Be careful to present positive aspects of services and benefits.

3. Be courteous to and considerate of everyone. It is easy, when asking for support from those who may not understand the needs and potential of persons who are visually impaired, to unintentionally reinforce incorrect attitudes of pity toward and concepts of helplessness about people who are blind. Often intense personal involvement or when there is frustration because of lack of support and understanding can lead to forgetting manners and letting anger control the situation. A proverb says "A soft word turneth away wrath." This is good to remember when conflicts arise or barriers prevent appropriate actions on behalf of those served.

4. Be able to understand others' viewpoints without blaming or judging. Understanding how otherS feel and think is crucial to good public relations. It is much more likely that support will be forthcoming when discussions and presentations are made that demonstrate a willingness to see the other side and to show that you value the opinions of others. This does not mean that one has to agree with or give up personal opinions. It usually means that there is still a gap in getting to a common understanding of the problems and issues.

DISCUSSION

As readers can see, the work of a professional working with individuals with visual impairments is not limited to teaching in the classroom or in the rehabilitation counselor's office. Perhaps with more than any other group of people, advocacy is needed. Very few people have an adequate and accurate understanding of what vision loss means. Most thinking people with visual disabilities do not want to be dependent on others, and want to be a positive force in their families and communities but, they are often prevented from becoming independent by attitudinal barriers and ignorance. Hence, the professional worker serving individuals with visual impairments needs far more than training as a teacher or counselor. Many aspects of the advocacy role of professionals in work for the blind must be taught more thoroughly in university training programs. One often knows what one needs to do in order to be an advocate without having it written into a job description. However, practicing advocacy skills needs to be part of a lifelong professional commitment.

SUGGESTED READINGS

1. Hadley School for the Blind. (1986). *Knowing the system.* Winnetka, IL: Hadley School.

Chapter 16

TRANSITION

INTRODUCTION

During the life span of individuals in most societies, there are points at which group expectations change. Social structures are often established to help meet the new expectations. After "rites of passage" or compliance with mores of an older group have been accomplished, the individual is accepted as an adult and is respected as an equal among other members of the society. The points at which changes in expectations are made are sometime referred to as transitions. Each society chooses its transition points. The common ones in the United States include infancy to preschool, preschool to kindergarten/elementary school, elementary school to secondary school, and from secondary school to postsecondary life that includes acquiring an occupation and assuming adult responsibilities. In recent years, more attention has been paid to transition points, especially the move from school to work by general education, special education, and vocational rehabilitation.

The aim of education is to prepare young people to take part in the life and continuity of their society. As societies have increased in complexity, so also has the formal education offered to the young to accomplish the aims in each society. In many Judeo-Christian societies a companion goal has been to maximize individual growth, with this goal seen as a contribution toward achieving societal goals. The value of the individual is the focus rather than only the society itself.

For many years, it has been observed that the modern Western societies have been deficient in the process by which children are assisted to make the transition from formal education to the adult role and also

167

for helping those who acquire disabilities to join society in full participation.

The change includes an extended period of adolescence and dependency and far too many of the young have failed to develop all the competencies necessary for meeting the needs of the broad adult society. Neither have they realized their own potential. This extended dependency has resulted from the greater affluence of industrial societies in comparison to more agrarian lives where children are considered as necessary and valued contributors to the welfare of the family and of society. Consequently, many young people in our society see life as meaningless and without a purpose, which has resulted in feelings of low self-esteem and worthlessness. Many adults who have been stricken with a disability face the same dependency and feelings of low self-worth.

The "baby boom" following World War II exacerbated the problem of transition and prolonged dependency because there has been a surplus of workers. This combined with the greater wealth of societies made it possible to provide for the needs of the society without making demands on the young or disabled to share in the burdens of providing for the economic needs of the family and the social group.

Those conditions of labor surplus and expanding wealth are rapidly changing as the "baby boomers" approach retirement. A large retired group has combined with a lowered birthrate to make it difficult for the active labor force to keep pace with economic demands. And, the increased use of the nation's wealth to support retired persons will place increased burdens on all who are or can be productive to assist in their support. At the same time, there is a push for the technically-sophisticated economy to require ever-higher levels of education for workers and there is a shrinkage in the number of jobs which can be performed with minimal training.

There is pressure to increase the size of the labor force. The abolition of the requirement that productive older persons be removed at age 65 from the labor force and into retirement is only one manifestation of this trend. Another is the reauthorization in 1990 of PL 101-336, the Americans with Disability Act (ADA), that has now brought the practices of discrimination against otherwise-potentially productive disabled persons into the picture. Society is beginning to recognize that it cannot afford to provide for those who are able to provide for themselves without lowering the standard of living for everyone else and from the viewpoint of the individuals involved who see themselves as second- or third-class citizens, all growth potential is severely limited unless unessential barriers are removed.

As an economy move, special-education services, which have been seen by many in the society as a convenient charitable means for caring for those with special problems, are being cut back. This "penny-wise, pound-foolish" approach means that those working with exceptional persons must do an increasingly difficult job with less resources allocated. If the efforts of special educators are not successful, the provisions of ADA will be relatively meaningless for those leaving the education system since these disabled persons will not be prepared to take advantage of the opportunities newly opened to them. Holding out the possibility for greater participation in society with one hand, while with the other, society reduces the rehabilitative and educational opportunities which will prepare disabled persons to accept these opportunities is doubly cruel since it will increase dependency when resources diminish and individuals with disabilities will not have the opportunity to grow and improve themselves.

Even though it is more difficult to properly prepare people with disabilities with restricted means, the effort must be made to educate the school-age population and rehabilitate adults with disabilities. The next challenge, though, is to help them build the bridge between school and the broader society, including the work place. As stated in the beginning of this chapter, this is known as "transition," and is the legacy of Madeline Will while she directed federal programs in vocational rehabilitation. From her own experience as the parent of a child with a disability, she recognized the barriers and, if nothing else, sensitized educators, rehabilitation programs, and prospective employers to the problem. Professionals are still involved in building the bridge of transition from school to work.

Visually impaired persons are, in many ways, more vulnerable to the pressures of present-day circumstances because their problems are so often misunderstood by the sighted world. Studies, as noted in an earlier chapter, have shown that the blind are viewed by prospective employers as being the most difficult to place in the work force. Perhaps that is part of the reason about two-thirds of the visually impaired who are "workforce eligible" and seeking employment across the nation are unemployed.

This chapter will consider transition and some of the factors which must be dealt with if it is to be successful. It will be particularly concerned with how professionals in field of work for the blind can help.

OBJECTIVES

Upon completing this chapter readers will be able to:

1. Identify and describe factors which are related to education, employment, and the transition between them.
2. Recognize barriers which limit persons with disabilities from participating fully in the life of their community.
3. Relate the growth of individuals to the welfare and progress of a society.
4. Develop plans for the successful transition of children and adults with visual impairments into the social and economic structure of their community.

IMPLEMENTING THE AMERICANS WITH DISABILITY ACT

The Americans with Disabilities Act of 1990 and its reauthorized versions provide the government's current attempt to prevent discrimination in the workplace. Reading the specific provisions of this very important piece of legislation with its accompanying regulations will provide information that will help professionals in special education and rehabilitation know what legal avenues are available for those with disabilities when they are faced with barriers to their employment and/or access to services. All professionals, as well as employers, should be aware of these provisions.

The Individuals with Disabilities Education Act (IDEA) also mandates activities to aid the transition of students from school to work. The regulations specify that beginning at age 14, planning teams must begin to have goals directed toward postsecondary outcomes. Students are invited to attend planning meetings and express their interests and select goals toward a time when they will transition from school to work and live as adults. Appropriate people from vocational rehabilitation services should also be present and help develop a rehabilitation plan, including training where necessary to reduce delays and keep individual students from "falling through the cracks" during the transition process.

Those who plan transition services for students with visual impairments are challenged by the diversity of the population. As pointed out in earlier chapters, vision loss is a very low incident population and there is a dramatic shortage of personnel trained to serve them. Thus, finding professionals knowledgeable enough about what it will take to establish a transition plan is difficult.

Further, the population of blind students includes a large proportion of individuals with disabilities in addition to sight loss. The needs of these students are vastly different from those who are able to leave school, perhaps further their education or training, and find their own living arrangements. Often a vast array of social services such as group homes, respite care for families, and medical issues must be a part of the transition planning.

Unlike those with other disabilities, in some states, there is no agency staffed and equipped to meet unique need of visually disabled students or adults. About half of the states attempt to meet the needs of the visually impaired with a "generic" rehabilitation service. In these "generic" programs, geographic location usually determines which counselor will serve the individual. Often these counselors have had minimal training regarding vision loss. A specialized service for the blind with staff who know the needs and have the skills to provide specific adaptive skills can offer a wider variety of options to the client who is blind.

CULTURAL CHANGE "THE THIRD WAVE"

In 1970, Alvin Toffler published his excellent book, *Future Shock* in which he discussed the shattering experience of too-rapid change upon a society He made the observation that Western society is experiencing rapid and dramatic changes in the lives of its citizens. He wrote a sequel entitled *The Third Wave,* in which he described the nature of the changes society is experiencing and provided a historical perspective. He suggested that the first economic wave, together with social context, consisted of the agrarian past during which each family was a unit. All of the needs of the family were met through the production of family members themselves or through barter between families. Crops and livestock provided food, with clothing coming from home production homespun cloth. Transportation was obtained from family livestock in the form of carts, wagons, carriages, and riding animals.

The second wave displaced this basic system with industrialization in which goods are produced through automated processes that were manned by people assembled in communities and individuals specialized in a specific task that contributed to the production which is then shared by all. Specialization allowed some to work in factories while others could distribute the products through commercial establishments while others provided services. No longer could each family produce all of the goods and services it needed. This wave has continued to expand and change until the present, though it is now in process of being replaced by the third wave, the "information revolution."

Toffler claims that society is well into the third wave where access to and possession of information is the basis for power. In the keynote address at a conference sponsored by the American Foundation for the Blind on the need for change in the services-delivery system for the visually impaired, he reiterated this theme and said that society stands on the threshold of this revolution. He cited changes in production from factory-produced items which are designed so "one size fits all" to individualization and customization of products. A good example of this is the current method for preparing eye glasses in the store which sells them rather than sending the individual's prescription out to a factory-like optical shop. He pointed out that clothing can now, in some places, be manufactured on site according to exact measurements and design preferences of the customer. No longer, he said, need the customers select from racks of clothing premade which never fit just right even with in-store alterations. The techniques involve "sewing" without sewing machines through heat-fusing processes which leave no seams.

He even went so far as to predict that in the very near future automobiles will be designed by the car salesman and the customer in the showroom on a computer with the design then transmitted by computer to the factory where parts would be ordered from the part-maker or the warehouse and assembled according to the design. Within a week the auto could be delivered, a one-of-a-kind vehicle.

He further suggested that much of the social upheaval now being experienced both locally and nationally are the result of the unsettling nature of these changes. While these changes hold great promise for individualization of the society to meet special needs, the same process is destabilizing to people caught in the backwash. This would be especially true for those who are not aware of the revolution and who are not prepared for it.

The application of these ideas to education and rehabilitation should be obvious, and important for those in special education and rehabilitation programs. Professionals cannot prepare their clients for specific jobs or even particular industries which are presently available because these jobs may not even be in existence when their clients enter the labor force. Just as cobblers, blacksmiths, and lamplighters, many of today's occupations will be replaced with technically more sophisticated employees, many of whom will be self-employed working out of their own homes. Computers and other electronic marvels will be available to allow remote access to employment. This shift of location will place a different emphasis on transportation, though not necessarily a lessened importance on accessing specific locations.

The key to accessing these new jobs will be proper preparation. But since professionals do not know what jobs will be available, how do they prepare clients for these jobs? The answer seems to lie in preparation in communication skills, flexibility, problem-solving, etc. which depend on utilization of information or knowledge which is available from remote information-storage systems.

While this sounds simple enough, it will be difficult to attain this kind of education in schools which are themselves like factories in which every effort is made to create a "finished product" which is largely indistinguishable from all others. If schools are to alter the rehabilitative and educational approach, professionals must learn how to individualize instruction, make it far more thought-provoking than at present and by providing training in interactive learning environments where "mastery" of subject matter is replaced by activities which have open-ended and multiple solutions for consideration.

If the aims and dreams of a society in which the disabled are able to be a fully-functioning PART of the emerging system, they must be prepared, along with the nondisabled, for a world which does not now exist. This will be especially challenging for the disabled since there will typically be less room for error. An "able body" and an "able mind" are more capable of making changes into unpredictable areas than for those with physical or mental problems which are generically restrictive. The same technological and informational explosion which has made it possible for the society to move into the information age will be the key to increasing the diversity of rehabilitative and educational opportunities which will, in turn, make it possible for the disabled individuals to participate more fully in the new world. But, while this dream of the future is unfolding, professionals must deal with the realities of the present.

ENABLING ENVIRONMENTS

As noted in the next chapter on "mainstreaming," there is a strong pressure to save money by forcing as many disabled students as possible into the regular classroom, even when this placement is, by nature, more restrictive than some separate facility which can offer the "most enabling environment." Professionals, as special educators, must go about the very difficult process of educating administrators to the fact that the individually-relevant rehabilitative and educational program for each student or client is the most appropriate model, not some arbitrarily selected "least restrictive environment." Though efficient and economical approaches are to be preferred, those goals should not be the determining criteria of an appropriate rehabilitative and educational opportunity. The current increase in activities by groups of persons with disabilities aimed at advocacy gives some ideas on the importance of dealing with this issue.

As discussed in Chapter 8, information access by large type, speech, and Braille are essential for children with vision loss if they are to be able to compete in meaningful rehabilitative and educational activities. The same is true for visually-impaired adults who seek to enter the labor force and to make career advancements once entry is achieved. If the changes predicted above by Toffler occur, reading and writing will become even more important requirements for participation in the information age. A minimum list of communication competencies would include print reading with or without special lenses and type enlargement; listening skills and ability to acquire materials on tape or through speech synthesis from computers; high-level computer literacy with additional technologies as CD ROM, flash memory card, database access, bulletin-board and other on-line access with a modem or DSL; laser discs, good keyboarding skills, Braille if print access is not good and/or if there is a poor prognosis for retaining residual vision; familiarity with visually-identified nonverbal cues, even if they cannot be observed directly so the visually-impaired can make appropriate use of such things as smiles, shrugs, facial expressions, and body movements; and, awareness of voice-transmitted emotional states.

If the visually-impaired youngster has speech, language, articulation, or voice defects, every effort should be made to have these corrected by appropriate therapy. Special emphasis should be placed on listening skills so the client can listen to compressed speech or other means for speeding up recorded materials. They should be taught how to use the several indexing methods currently in use in order to be able to locate information on tapes or discs quickly and easily.

The terms "looking," "seeing," and "reading" all refer to the use of the eyes, but have different connotations. There are no comparable terms for differences in hearing processes, though "hearing" and "listening" imply slightly different uses of the ears. In particular, some educators have noted the absence of a term which corresponds to the visual term "reading" and have suggested the term "auding" to correspond to that visual process for getting information. It is instructive to note that, whereas reading is taught as an integral part of the elementary-school curriculum throughout all grades, there is little training provided for "auding." It is also instructive to note that numerous studies have shown that children below the sixth grade typically learn more through listening than from visual presentations, and this in spite of the above-mentioned lack of training. This seems to imply that for all children, but especially for those with vision loss, systematic and consistent training in the development of auding skills should be provided. There is no justification for assuming auding skills will develop in all children without help.

In most states, special education and rehabilitation services are provided by two separate agencies. In earlier times, this was necessary because of federal funding patterns. As a consequence, there was often little contact between these two agencies, and there was virtually no planning for the transition of disabled children into adult life. Laws and regulations that set 16 years as the age at which rehabilitation services could be offered made the natural separation between schools and adult services even more distant than they needed to be. Recently, however, the age floor was lowered to age 14 years and cooperative agreements have been set up to make transition easier. Planning prior to age 14 is possible on the part of the rehabilitation agency, though no funds can be spent prior to that age. Some jurisdictions make all school data on disabled children available on a routine basis from the schools.

Some rehabilitation agencies currently have both rehabilitation teachers and rehabilitation counselors assigned so as to cover the entire state. Services may also be provided at a center for the blind for young children who are nearing the end of their basic rehabilitative and educational programs. These activities include mobility and daily-living programs, personal and family counseling, career days, work experiences, and equipment demonstrations.

Many regular classroom teachers, school administrators, and guidance counselors are not aware of some of the services offered to persons with vision impairments. This is especially true in rural areas, and, therefore, professional in work for the blind are encouraged to share what they have learned about transition with these educators. They will undoubtedly get a varied reaction from these professionals because they will share in the range of attitudes held by the public at large about the visually impaired. This example should provide those who work with the blind with a great incentive to broaden their understanding, not by stepping on their toes, but by sensitizing them to the problems and potentials of the blind.

EMPLOYMENT BARRIERS TO THE DISABLED

Little has been said about one of the most important parts of the transition team, e.g., employers and potential employers. Although there are strong incentives for employers to hire disabled workers, there is often great reluctance to do this. There are many misconceptions about disabled workers, especially those with disabilities related to vision. One such misconception is that insurance rates increase when disabled workers are employed. Studies have shown that disabled workers have better-than-average records in such matters as being on time, reduced absenteeism, and in productivity. Insurance rates do not rise when hiring disabled workers, especially when these workers are properly trained, suitably placed, and REGULARLY monitored for performance over time by the rehabilitation agency.

As mentioned earlier in this chapter, PL 101–336 deals with a requirement that employers—with a few exceptions—cannot discriminate in hiring practices, training programs, and promotions on the basis of disability. Even on their application forms or during interviews, they cannot ask questions about the applicant's physical or mental conditions. They must also make reasonable accommodations to facilitate adequate job performance by disabled workers, and necessary training and equipment must be provided under most circumstances.

Unless the disabled person is capable of performing the duties and assuming the responsibilities under these conditions, the employer is not obligated to hire, train, or retrain them. As noted above, this is reason to foster and encourage adequate rehabilitative and educational provisions for persons with disabilities. Penalties and/or incentives will never completely break down the barriers or take the place of properly prepared persons with disabilities who are capable of and willing to make a meaningful contribution toward achieving the goals of employers.

SUCCESSFUL BLIND PERSONS

In the early 1930s, Louise Wilber, herself blind, wrote her doctoral dissertation on vocational guidance for the visually impaired. She found examples of blind individuals successful in a wide range of occupations ranging from professions to construction to service delivery. This indicated to her that blindness, per se, should not pose a barrier to most occupations. The fact that those without sight could perform the tasks involved in a particular job, therefore, proved that something other than sight loss determined whether one was successful or not in a chosen field.

Since that time studies conducted by vocational rehabilitation agencies have amply confirmed her findings and conclusions with examples of blind individuals serving in positions such as United States Senator, Attorney General for a state, electrical engineer, business executive, psychiatrist, carpenter, auto mechanic, chicken farmer, service-station attendant, etc., etc., etc. With the exception of occupations that specifically require eyesight—pilot, taxi driver, surgeon, for example—there seems to be no limit to vocations in which blind persons have been successful. "Where there is a will, there is a way." The jobs are not performed in the same way a sighted person would do the task, but ingenious ways have been found that enable one without sight to perform the task.

One of the authors associated with a man who had worked for many years as an auto tune-up mechanic for a national chain. He lost his sight as the result of a battery blowing up in his face, and destroying his corneas. With the assistance of his family, his neighbors, and vocational rehabilitation, he built a garage behind his home and equipped it with the latest in test equipment. His wife, who was a homemaker, would come out to the shop when he needed dials read, then return to her chores. He would take starters and alternators apart and rebuild them, replace spark plugs, replace wiring harnesses, adjust and rebuild carburetors, etc. using his fingers and tools and only occasionally needing his wife's eyes. He had the reputation as the best tune-up man in his medium-sized city and many of the companies who had used the services while he was employed by the national chain moved their business to him in his new shop. He was far more successful financially in his own business than he had been working for someone else.

The same author also knew a man who had been an officer in the Mexican Army, had left that to become a chef on several of the great ocean liners then used for world tours, and then lost his sight. After a period of adjustment, he resumed his gourmet cooking for a small restaurant.

In both of these cases, the person had learned his vocation before losing his sight, and then was able to devise means for performing the same tasks in a modified manner. There are many other individuals who entered training for their occupation after losing eyesight.

Thomas Bentham was born blind, but had a strong interest in science, especially in engineering. He received his doctorate in electrical engineering and successfully taught this subject at Haverford College in Haverford, Pennsylvania. He used his knowledge to modify equipment so it could be used by people without sight, making them available through a company he founded, Science for the Blind, Inc. He was instrumental in the development of the laser cane, a device presently used by some blind persons as their primary travel aid.

It might appear that successful persons without sight are the rare geniuses, but that the run-of-the-mill blind could not succeed at any kind of highly technical trade or profession, and even if they succeeded in obtaining training, they would not be able to ply their trade. Based on this assumption, a number of professions have set up criteria for admission to training which systematically exclude those without sight. In Great Britain, the occupation of a physical therapist has been designated for special training for the blind, while in this country the blind are excluded from following in this profession. The authors have known individuals who were trained in this occupation and successfully practiced it who would be excluded in today's world. The practice of osteopathy is another example. The authors were acquainted with two men who had long and successful careers in osteopathic medicine before the blind were excluded from the training.

There is a national organization for blind teachers with several hundred members who are attempting to open more teaching positions for young blind persons wishing to pursue a career in education. While there is no blatant policy which excludes visually-impaired persons from training in this profession, most training programs are so structured, with rigid requirements that require sight, that it is very difficult for one without sight to succeed in the training. And, even when they have successfully navigated through the training program, it is extremely difficult to obtain employment. Administrators cannot understand how they (the administrators) could perform their duties without sight, and are, therefore, convinced that a blind person could not perform them either.

Those who practice this form of subtle discrimination are not evil, unfeeling persons; they are simply misguided and misinformed. But their influence upon visually impaired persons is negative and reduces their potential for success. Their predictions of failure become self-fulfilling prophecies. It is, indeed, the rare blind person who is willing to proceed to prepare for and enter upon a vocation in which he or she has been excluded because of discrimination and to successfully negotiate the minefield of prejudice to a successful vocational destination.

Experience with other types of anti-discrimination laws suggests that the ADA will not solve the problem overnight. This type of legislation may help to open some doors and to remove some obvious barriers, but unless and until visually-impaired persons prepare themselves to take advantage of the new opportunities, and demonstrate that they can successfully perform, all of the psychological barriers will not come down. The playing field can be made more nearly level, but the disabled still must compete on that field before acceptance and respect will be won.

Professionals can determine for themselves the validity of the above-described situation by selecting a person in their community who is successful in his/her chosen vocation. Arrange an interview with this person and ask him/her about the possibility of a person with limited sight successfully COMPETING in that occupation. Explore with this person the specific tasks which might prove most difficult to perform with limited or no sight, and then go on to explore ways in which the tasks could be performed.

DISCUSSION

In the process of transition for visually impaired persons, our profession must "make haste slowly." Professionals have essentially two tasks: first, they must prepare those with whom they work to prepare themselves psychologically, physically, socially, and vocationally so they can, in fact, succeed in an occupation if they have the chance; and, second, they must help change misguided public attitudes which would exclude from the field those who can succeed. People are people, and it cannot be expected—short of the millennium—to create a perfect society, but professionals can work with those for whom they have responsibility so that they enhance their chances for success. As someone has rightly observed, "it is better to light one little candle than to curse the darkness."

The last chapter of this book will deal with the issue of whether there is a need for a "psychology of blindness." Sentiments on this issue change with alterations in the Zeitgeist or World View of a given time. The current Zeitgeist, as we have noted, is dominated by a nomothetic, generic mentality which would hold that there is no need for specializations. In a former time, the need to understand individuals would have held that there is a need for specialized understandings for specific disability groups. The "third wave" indicates that perhaps a return to specialization is needed. The authors will not resolve the issue, but perhaps they will be able to help readers make an informed choice.

SUGGESTED READINGS

1. Bauman, M.K. (1966). *Adjustment to blindness reviewed.* Springfield, IL: Charles C Thomas.
2. Toffler, A. (1974). *Future shock—Learning for tomorrow: The roll of the future in education.* New York: Random House.
3. Toffler, A. (1980). *The third wave.* New York: Morrow.
4. Wilber, L. (1937). *Vocations for the visually handicapped.* Oxford: American Foundation for the Blind.

Chapter 17

MAINSTREAMING

INTRODUCTION

In 1975, the Congress of the United States passed PL 94–142, the Education of All Handicapped Children Act. This law provided that all children with handicaps are entitled to a free appropriate public education in the least restrictive environment. The law was re-authorized in 1990, 1997, and 2004 with the title of Individuals with Disabilities Education Act (IDEA).

Although these laws are generally viewed as major milestones in the advancement of education of exceptional children, many questions remain to be answered about aspects of their educational provisions and, more particularly, about the rules and regulations supporting them. Most of these questions center about the double negative term, "least restrictive environment (LRE)."

At the national level, the LRE has generally been interpreted to mean in an education setting along with nondisabled peers and within the local or neighborhood school. Critics have suggested the need to substitute the double positive term, "most enabling environment (MEE) for the LRE. It is claimed that this term carries the idea that each child's education should take place in a setting selected from a variety of options which are designed to maximize educational opportunities.

The term used most to defend where and how education services are to be provided is appropriate. The term appropriate avoids the double negative, but it does not emphasize the postitive. Many view use of the term appropriate as the result of the Rowley v. (see Suggested Reading #2. Board of Education v. Rowley, 1982) in which the Supreme Court of the United States decided it was not necessary to provide an education that would assure that students with disabilities would reach their highest potential but that the education provided must be appropriate. Many court decisions and due process hearings have tried to establish what "appropriate" means. Each court has ultimately looked to the facts of an individual situation in making its decision which at least might meet the intent of the word "individual" in the original legislations.

The major problem in using any of these terms is how to describe an array of elements in a continuum of services together with the parts of each element which make the most meaningful contribution to a child's education. It is further argued that the appropriate placement along the continuum of services will not only differ for each child, but will vary for each group of children with common, educationally relevant characteristics including any specific disability. Thus, the range of services for the developmentally young child would probably be quite different than for a child with hearing impairments, one with visual impairments, or one with a learning disability.

The ultimate goal of special educational services is to prepare for integration of exceptional children into the broader society to the maximum extent possible. Subgoals which contribute to this major goal are such factors as development of an accurate self concept, creation of high self esteem, teaching and development of vocational skills, expectations of high academic achievement, training in consistent work habits, etc. Other contributing factors which lie outside the control of the schools are such things as public attitudes toward the disabled, provisions for vocational rehabilitation, availability of appropriate living arrangements, opportunities for social interactions including marriage, health care, etc.

Those who advocate the inclusion of all disabled children in local, neighborhood schools argue that the schools are a model or prototype of the society as a whole. While this idea is attractive, it flies in the face of facts.

Among the characteristics of the public school system which differ significantly from the broader society are the following:

1. Students are not employed by private-sector businesses, nor are they self-employed or self-supporting.

2. Schools are not democratic institutions, at all levels of administration but are far more like totalitarian or welfare governments than the government of the United States.

3. Nondisabled students often resent the special provisions for disabled students, and develop nonpositive attitudes toward the disabled.

4. Families are an integral part of the broader society, but in schools, there are no groupings which resemble family units.

5. Even with assistance that disabled children receive, there are extremely large differences in the academic achievement among the diverse groupings of disabled and nondisabled students. Although the same differences of ability exist in the society at large, they are not so obvious because of the differences in living arrangements. Also, special considerations for low performance due to a disability are far less available in the world outside of schools.

A number of studies have been conducted which shed light on some of the components in the array of services which society provides to achieve the major goal of mainstreaming. However, much more research remains to be done, and quality answers to questions about what aspects of the program need to be modified must be provided before intelligent decisions can be made.

Children with visual handicaps and adults without sight provide unique groups for studying some aspects of the problem. Long before the current programs for special education mandated by PL 94–142 in 1975, the field of vision impairments had developed an array of services and has had over a century of experience with some of these.

Residential schools for children without sight were established in this country as early as 1829. Segregated classrooms in regular schools were started in 1900. Integrated programs with children with visual impairments attending most classes with sighted compatriots and "pulled out" for special help in a resource room or by an itinerant teacher have been operating in some places since before World War II. Vocational rehabilitation services have been available in programs which service all disability groups and in separate agencies serving the blind since 1943. And, these variations have existed in parallel settings as well as in holistic, statewide programs.

During the decades of the 1950s and 1960s, a major shift in where children with visual handicaps were educated took place. Hapeman discovered the changes created considerable friction between proponents favoring an integrated program and those who believed a residential option gained better overall results. Out of this conflict came research which dealt with some outcomes of these two broad approaches. For example, educational achievement was studied. Self-concept and self-esteem were studied by Head. Social adjustment was studied by Crandell and Streeter. These studies are only representative of many others which dealt with these and other aspects of education of the visually impaired.

This chapter will look at the issue of where children with visual handicaps should be educated. It will also consider evidence concerning the benefits derived from each of the options presently available.

OBJECTIVES

At the completion of this chapter te reader will be able to:

1. Describe the three most frequently used options for the education of children with visual handicaps, together with the benefits claimed for each of these options.
2. Evaluate the needs of children with visual handicaps and describe how these needs can be provided most effectively and efficiently.
3. Discuss the adequacy of present educational options for meeting the needs of children with visual impairments necessary for eventual integration into the societal mainstream as adults.
4. Act as an advocate for children with visual handicaps in the schools, in the community, and before decision makers.

COMMON EDUCATION PATTERNS

Readers are invited now to consider the three most common types of service delivery which have been developed for children with visual impairments: residential schools, resource rooms, and itinerant services. Consider also the educational needs of children with visual disabilities—both needs which are common to all children and needs which reflect special problems of this group of students. Next, consider the likelihood that each of these various needs will be met in one of the educational service delivery systems mentioned above. On the basis of this analysis, what would one conclude about which approach is best, if there is, in fact, a best approach? A brief description of each major option for educating children with visual impairments will follow.

However, before beginning the program description, a brief description, of the population of visually impaired students is in order. It should be kept in mind that visual impairment is a very low incident population in schools. Estimates range from 1–2/1,000 school-age children. National estimates support a figure of about 95,000 in the total school-age population of near 44 million. These numbers include a very heterogenous groups whose visual abilities range from total absence of sight to the ability to read regular size print with the aid of enlargement or holding pages very close. The instructional media may be Braille, print, audio recordings, or a combination. And, it must be remembered that subject matter and ages range from preschool through secondary school. Teachers and other professionals such as orientation and mobilty instructors must master both subject area content as well as the adaptive methods needed for each student. Finally, as medical advances save more and younger premature babies, many children have disabilities in addition to blindness including cortical visual impairments.

Residential Schools

The most widely used model of service until the 1960s was the residential school. It should be noted that the term residential referred only to the addition of facilities to provide board and room for students who lived too far from a central campus to travel home on a daily basis. Instruction generally followed the state prescribed curriculum. However, because of the expense and shortage of Braille and large print materials, texts were generally selected from those produced by the American Printing House for the Blind (APH). A part of the training included daily living skills that were practiced in the dormitories. Vocational training was also available in many schools. Extracurricular activities were also an important part of the education program.

Most schools participated in interscholastic sports, debate, music, Boy/Girl Scouts, along with school sponsored dances, dramatics, camping, field trips, etc. Proponents of a residential school education emphasized that full-time staff were available in all aspects of the program by creating a critical mass of students. This allows more attention to be given to the unique needs of students with visual impairments, including skills of daily living and socal skills, etc. They also point out the cost savings of sharing equipment and materials.

Resource Rooms

Like residential programs, resource rooms were established when there was a sufficient number of students at a close age range.in a local community. Students are bused to a central school location on a daily basis. Where possible children were grouped according to age and classroom space was provided in a preschool, elementary, junior high, or high school.

Generally these settings used the same curriculum prescribed by the state and if possible texts and materials were the same as in the school where classes were located. The resource classroom room was provided with special equipment needed for instruction and a trained teacher of the visually impaired assisted students and teachers within the school to meet the academic needs of the students. Many dedicated resource room teachers also made certain that their students were included in the extracurricular programs of the school.

Students might spend all or only part of their day in the resource room. At the end of the day, students were transported to their homes. Parents were responsible for daily living skills. Additional transportation was needed when students participated in extracurricular or social activities with students from the school where the resource room was located.

Itinerant Services

Where an itinerant service is used, students with visual impairment usually attend classes in their neighborhood school. As with other models, the state curriculum is used and the texts and materials used in the school are the same as for other students in the school. Often, the student served by the itinerant teacher may be the only person with a severe visual impairment in the school. The itinerant teacher visits the school on a regular basis to provide help to the student and the regular classroom teacher(s).

Adaptive texts, materials, and equipment are brought from resource centers or purchased by the school. Sometimes these things are loaned from state education resource centers or textbook depositories.

When the itinerant teacher visits a school, he/she may consult with the teacher(s) and make arrangements to provide special materials; consult with the student to identify areas needing assistance; provide special training in specific academic areas with the use of adapted materials or equipment; or provide instruction in adaptive skills such as Braille, orientation and mobility and daily living skills.

Many itinerant teachers also make certain that opportunities to participate in elective classes and extracurricular sports and activities are provided. Since students attend school in their neighborhood schools, they live at home and daily transportation is provided in the same way as for all students in the school.

ADVANTAGES AND DISADVANTAGES

Now, consider some of the claimed advantages and disadvantages for these three settings:

Residential School (Advantages)

1. Materials and equipment especially designed for children with visual handicaps are available. The same materials and equipment can be used by successive groups of children.
2. All teachers would be specialists in the education of children with visual handicaps. In service programs are more easily and specifically designed for these specialists.
3. There is less likelihood that problems observed in only one or two children will be considered as characteristics of children with visual handicaps since they could be seen against the backdrop of many children with visual handicaps.
4. In like manner, individual needs would be seen in contrast to the needs of the overall group of children with visual handicaps.
5. Programs and curricula can be designed with the needs of children with visual handicaps in mind. Physical education, music, reading, mobility, typing for younger children, word processing, vocational classes, etc. can be especially geared to meet special and unique needs.

Residential School Disadvantages

1. Children are taken out of the home at an early age and lose the shaping influence of parents and siblings.
2. It is more expensive since the program adds room and board and 24-hour-a-day supervision.
3. Children have fewer opportunities to associate with their peers who are sighted.
4. Because the total enrollment at the secondary level is small, few elective courses can be offered on campus in subjects such as foreign languages, higher math, science, etc.

Resource Room Advantages

1. Children with visual handicaps are often in regular classes with children with sight and with regular teachers for at least part of the day.
2. Children receive specific help in areas such as Braille, mobility, remedial subjects, etc.
3. It is far less expensive than residential schools.
4. Some specialized materials and equipment can be maintained on site.
5. Progress of the child with visual handicaps is compared to sighted peers rather than with others with similar problems.

Resource Room Disadvantages

1. Since only one or a very small number of children in most neighborhood schools are visually impaired, they must be transported from neighborhood schools to some centralized location.
2. Seldom can specialized curricula and programs be provided just for children with visual handicaps.
3. Materials and equipment used by one child may not be needed for other children with visual handicaps. This often means that these materials and pieces of equipment are either stored or disposed of.

Itinerant Programs Advantages

1. Children can live at home and attend neighborhood schools with their neighbors.

2. This is less expensive than residential schools or resource rooms.
3. Children with visual handicaps are in the regular classroom and specialized help is provided for both the regular teacher and other specialists.

Itinerant Programs Disadvantages

1. Only limited access to specialized services, programs, equipment, and materials is available. Teacher specialists cannot transport all that is needed. Mobility, music and physical education are provided on a limited basis.
2. The progress of the child with visual handicaps is compared with that of children with sight exclusively.
3. The child with visual handicaps is seldom, if ever, given the opportunity to learn special adaptive skills from others who have mastered them. In other words, he/she lacks role models for living as children with visual handicaps in a sighted world.
4. The child with visual handicaps often becomes a "mascot" for students with normal vision and his/her teacher and is seldom considered as a normal, fully functioning member of the class and accepted as a part of the school.
5. A major portion of teacher time is spent in travel from school to school.

Godfrey Stevens clarification of the meanings of the terms "impairment," "disability," and "handicap" as discussed below.. Note particularly the extended definitions of the areas of "handicap" as described by Stevens. These extensions are needed to reflect the idea of burdens which distinguish exceptional children from their nonexceptional peers, i.e., mobility, communications (reading and writing, etc), social interactions, concept formation and transition to employment.

Both in the fields of special education and vocational rehabilitation, the terms "impairment," "disability," and "handicap" are often used interchangeably even though they have quite different origins. The correct use of these terms could aid in clarifying the problems in programs for the subjects of rehabilitation and special education.

Impairment is a medical term and refers to diseased, disordered, or missing body-organ tissues. The defect in the tissues may be derived from heredity, injury, or organ inactivity. The brain dysfunction in

Mongolism is caused by defects in the RNA from the time of conception of the child. Baldness is an impairment, and often comes from one's family background. Injuries can result in organ loss as in amputations, surgical removals, or scar development. Body-organ tissues may deteriorate if they are not used regularly. Exercise, improper eating habits, and old age can produce impairments.

The term "disability" is the negation of the term "able." Each body organ performs one or more specific tasks or functions. If the organ does not perform these tasks or functions, either because of impairments or because these tasks and functions have not been learned, a disability exists.

Which of the settings listed above would best be equipped to reduce these handicaps? The answer to this question must take into account the lifetime perspective, i.e., are the handicaps an impediment to participation in the broader society when children become adults? It is not just a matter of surviving in a limited school environment.

FULL INCLUSION

The debate over which type of services are best is likely to continue for some time. However, it is hoped that personal philosophy would not overrule sound practices. It is plain that each model of service has some advantages and disadvantages. Given the diversity of the population, all the models are probably appropriate at least for some children. It is also likely that each model could serve an individual child at some point during his/her education. Expecting one model to meet the needs of all children with visual impairments throughout his/her life is perhaps letting philosophy or economics limit the potential of the student.

As noted in the introduction, the present Zeitgeist in the United States strongly supports educating all disabled students (including those with visual disabilities) in the regular classroom. If not validated as appropriate, then this approach is probably "penny wise and pound foolish." This model of services is nevertheless a matter of reality. But, if professionals consider carefully the special needs of the visually impaired, better ways must be found to provide the kinds and quality of services that are appropriate to the person, regardless of setting.

DISCUSSION

It seems clear that the present emphasis on mainstreaming is based on economic considerations, and this addresses only immediate concerns rather than long-term considerations for success of children with visual impairments. Professionals in this field, of course, need to do more research to understand the consequences which follow from specific educational approaches. But results in hand, from research, point to major costs to society which will become even higher unless effective and efficient educational programs are developed. For example, of the nation's adults with no sight who are labor force eligible (i.e., are between the ages of 18 and 65 years, with no disabling conditions beyond vision loss and who are actively seeking employment), 67 percent are unemployed. That figure is roughly ten times the percentage rate for the population as a whole. This means that families or society must be taking care of the unemployed. Even though children with visual handicaps constitute a relatively small group, can society afford that continual economic drain? And, that says nothing about the sheer waste of human talents and abilities.

SUGGESTED READINGS

1. Bishop, V.E. (2004). *Teaching visually impaired children* (3rd ed.). Springfield, IL: Charles C Thomas.
2. Board of Education of the Hendrick Hudson Central School District, Westchester County et al. v. Rowley by her Parents Rowley et.us. U.S. Supreme Court No. 80–1002 June 28, 1982.
3. Thomas, G.E. (1992). *Mainstreaming, Are there any ill effects?* unpublished paper. Brigham Young University, Provo, UT.

Chapter 18

PSYCHOLOGY OF BLINDNESS

INTRODUCTION

Psychology has been subdivided into a number of related areas of specialization including industrial psychology, clinical psychology, social psychology, and rehabilitative and educational psychology. Each of these specializations has been further subdivided into smaller, more compact areas. For example, rehabilitative and educational psychology have been divided into counseling psychology, instructional psychologies, psychology of exceptional children, school psychology, etc. Textbooks for each of the subdivisions could be cited as examples of these. William Croockshank, for an example, edited a text entitled *Psychology of Exceptional Children and Youth*, which was used in courses many years ago.

Samuel P. Hayes, during the 1940s, wrote a book entitled *Toward a Psycholgy of Blindness*, which is no longer in print. The book detailed some aspects of blindness which Dr. Hayes considered to require a specialized treatment which was not available in more general areas of psychology, for example, the so-called sixth sense of the blind, intellectual abilities of the blind, academic achievement, etc.

Still later, a journal was published in Japan with the name of *Psychology of the Blind*. It reported about research which dealt with the blind, but since it was printed in Japanese, it is difficult to identify specifically the kinds of materials included between its covers.

Behaviorism, as a distinct theory, developed during the 1920s with the work of John B. Watson and Edward L. Thorndike as major contributors in this country and Ivan Pavlov in Russia. Its proponents did not consider behaviorism as an example of psychological theory, but as an application of scientific methodology to the study of behavior change. This approach rejected as essentially unscientific methods and topics then in wide use by psychologists such as introspection, synthesis, memory, and personality analysis with projectile devices. These approaches were rejected because their research foci were not directly observable. Behaviorists chose to accept that only those things which can be observed, measured, and quantified came within the purview of science, it was claimed. Psychology was not the study of the mind or soul, intentions, volitions, thoughts, feelings, aspirations, neuroses, psyche, not even brain processes because these could be only inferred. Someone observed that at the time of the development of behaviorism, psychology lost its mind and then lost consciousness, conditions from which it has never fully recovered.

Under the onslaught of behaviorism, the different fields of psychology came into disrepute. Few of them survived. The psychology of blindness, which was developing under Cruickshank, Hayes, Cholden, Cutsforth, and others was "biting the dust," along with others. The impact of blindness, it was argued, had no "meaning" beyond changes in behavior which could be the only basis for a new understanding only achievable through behavioral psychology–the study of behavior.

Not all psychologists agreed with this radical empirical approach, and continued to work within other divisions of psychology. The American Psychological Association continued to recognize the divisions in its organizational structure and as the behavioral approach began to wane in the last decade or two, the divisions have been revitalized and prospered.

The premise of this book has been to suggest it is time to consider reviving the study of the special problems, needs, characteristics, and treatment of those with vision loss. Earlier chapters have pointed out that growth and development, cognitive processes, mobility difficulties, etc. may share aspects of other divisions of psychology, education, and rehabilitation but that the unique aspects of blindness justify the special focus that could come from studies based on a psychology of blindness.

The focus of this chapter will be on some of the issues which have been covered in previous chapters as they might contribute to a better understanding of human beings in general. The bias which generates this chapter should be obvious, but there is no intention of forcing acceptance of that bias.

OBJECTIVES

Upon completion of this chapter readers will be able to:

1. Identify and discuss some of the unique characteristics of a study of vision loss.
2. Recognize how these unique characteristics might shed light on broader issues in psychology.
3. Consider potential research topics that could clarify some of the issues included here.
4. Describe other biases than the one included here that might be used to counter the proposed development of a psychology of blindness.

THERE ARE NO TWO ALIKE

Consider the following ideas. Perhaps the reason Lowenfeld's observation that, other than vision loss, there are no characteristics which are shared by all of the visually impaired is valid because the concept of blindness is disjunctive rather than conjunctive. It is commonly understood that this group can be subdivided into many subgroups on such bases as those with varying amounts of vision, the age of the onset of vision loss, the duration, the cause of vision loss, amount and types of rehabilitation and education acquired, etc., which means that there is no set of attributes, qualities, characteristics, properties, or traits that can be inferred from membership in the category, Visually Impaired. But there is reason to believe that exemplars of some of the subcategories which would be derived from an analysis of the disjunctive concept would share common characteristics beyond those used to specifically define them. For example, Stephens and Simpkins, in their study of the cognitive functioning of the blind compared to the sighted, found that there was a major deficit on almost all of the 29 subtests used. Even though it was found that deficits could be remediated save for the deficit in spatial concepts the fact that these blind children shared some underlying qualities which put them at risk is important. If nothing else, it showed that specialized or additional instructional approaches were required for their subjects to attain normal functioning. Neither the modifications in the testing equipment and materials nor remedial approaches needed by the blind were required for normally seeing children. The use of special materials and procedures was needed for the blind children alone.

There is some anecdotal evidence available which suggests that even for subjects who are totally blind, differences related to the onset of blindness are meaningful and identifiable. Children who are blind from birth have more difficulty in spatial orientation than those who lost sight after an initial sighted period. With one exception, it has yet to be shown that any of the congenitally blind are without some deficit in spatial orientation. The one possible exception to this surmise comes from children who are blind because of congenital, bilateral retinoblastoma in which both eyes must be removed in order to save the child's life from the cancer. There is some anecdotal evidence that this group is much superior in spatial orientation to even later blinded children. The cancer is genetically transmitted, according to the research of David Kitchens of the Columbia Presbyterian Medical Center in New York City. As a group, they differ in intelligence from their siblings who do not carry the gene, scoring on average 10 IQ points higher. This does not, for the most part, negate the observation concerning the need for blind persons to have had some sight before they can develop normal spatial orientation. Rather, it suggests that there is partial genetic compensation for this one group of blind persons.

It is not likely that hypotheses which can be derived from the above discussed observations will be develop and pursued by anyone who is only interested in solution that affect more people or solve more general problems. They are, rather, the kinds of hypotheses which someone in the area of psychology of blindness might want to investigate. If these questions are important, then a psychology of blindness with personnel trained at graduate levels in this discipline will be needed in order to get the research conducted.

SUPPORT FOR A PSYCHOLOGY OF BLINDNESS

A psychiatrically-oriented researcher, Selma Fraiberg, has studied developmental patterns in blind children as they interact with the environment, and has found deviations in those patterns from patterns found in normal children. Her observations were conducted on limited numbers of blind children, but they point to some possible direct effects of vision loss on developmental processes. Even if one were to argue that the differences may be remediated, the fact that the patterns differ, as a consequence of vision loss, is significant and would warrant investigation by a psychologist studying blindness. Such inquiries could possibly lead to information that would be useful in establishing better instruction and training methods for blind as well as sighted children.

As noted in earlier chapters, Verna Hart at the University of Pittsburgh found that blind babies avoid the prone position, an avoidance which inhibits their development in crawling and exploring. The blind may possess all of the physiological and psychological characteristics necessary for moving and searching, but the blindness itself prevents these processes from guiding the development of the child. Again, this supports the need for specialization in blindness per se in order to explore the ramifications of such observations.

As a matter of fact, David Warren's excellent book, *Blindness and Early Childhood Development,* is replete with examples of factors which appear to be influenced by vision loss. It also describes the wide range of research and findings which has characterized work with the blind. Although a background in normal childhood development is essential for interpreting this mass of data, it again argues for the need for continued specialization in this area. For the general developmental psychologist, these data may be interesting and suggest factors in normal development that are worth investigating, but the full implications of this work will likely be of no vital importance except to the psychologist studying blindness.

In traditional scientific inquiry methods, all variables possible are held constant so changes in one variable, the independent variable, can be studied to see what effects these changes have on the dependent or outcome variable(s). It would be desirable, were it possible, to make certain that no other factor, including chance variations, could have produced the results of the study. To the extent that extraneous variables are controlled, the study is thought to be valid. Animal studies, where some controls are permitted that could not be controlled with humans, sometime suggest that blindness imposes a different way of operating in order for the blind to perform.

In a study conducted by David Krech and his associates at the University of California at Berkeley, a litter of rats was randomly divided into two groups. Rats in one group were blinded and those in the other were not. The two groups were then reared as nearly in the same manner as possible. At maturity both groups of rats were taught to run an elevated maze. When all had learned the task to a criterion level, all were sacrificed and parts of their brains examined. The sighted rats had visual cortices which were significantly larger and heavier than the blind rats. The blind rats had somothetic cortices which were significantly larger and heavier than the sighted rats. The presence or absence of sight produced highly significant differences in brain structures, and, hence, most likely to psychological processes as well. The number of neurons or nerve cells did not differ, but the number and size of glial or supporting cells differed for the brain areas studied.

A study such as this would not have been possible with human subjects, but there is always a problem in extrapolating from lower organisms to higher.

Lee Robinson, in his doctoral research, noted a relatively large number of dissertations which he had examined were conducted on visually impaired subjects. Most of the studies were done by individuals who did not work in the blindness field, but this observation seems to reflect the recognition on the part of some researchers that blind children, to the extent they are typical of the general population, offer an interesting control variable. A psychology of blindness would gather and evaluate such studies for ideas which could drive the education and rehabilitation efforts. David Warren, cited above, using this proposed approach, demonstrated what could be done with a blindness research focus.

SOCIOLOGY OF BLINDNESS

Many professionals in work for the blind, especially those who work with young children, are familiar with *Growing Up: A Developmental Curriculum*, the *Oregon Project*, and/or the *Hawaii Early Leaning Profile*. These programs, along with others, were developed to study and guide developmental progress and have been used extensively with visually impaired children from birth to about age six. Preliminary data indicate that the developmental profiles which can be generated can differentiate areas of differences for different disability groups as well as for individuals within a group who have special problems. *Growing Up*, for example, profiles development along 51 strands in six broad areas of growth–fine motor, cognitive, self care, physical, speech and language, and social. As a research framework, this approach could identify differences in patterns for infants and small children that could lead to more intensive study and potentially to better interventions to assist children with disabilities to grow normally.

A difficulty in researching these areas related to blindness, as well as any others, is finding enough subjects with a similar set of characteristics in order to make any findings statistically significant. Research literature submitted to the professional journals is replete with studies but virtually always has such small samples that generalizations cannot be made with any degree of confidence. In the 1960s, efforts were made to collect basic data for national comparison using a Model Reporting Area. This project was discontinued due to lack of funding, or interest by the general fields of education and rehabilitation, along with the usual difficulties of design and maintenance of a large data base.

A new effort has been made by the American Printing House for the Blind (APH). The goal is to develop a national data base for children with visual impairments ages birth to three years old that can be used by APH to analyze trends of children coming into the education system and using the information determining products that will be of most use to schools. It would be a major benefit to the field if a broader age range were maintained. Such a source that included even basic demographics could allow for identification and selection of samples large enough for statistically significant research studies.

PSYCHOLOGY OF BLINDNESS

With the aid of new techniques, neuro psychologists are beginning to map the regions of the human brain and the functions they perform during normal psychological activities. This research seems to indicate that psychological processes are far more complex than had been imagined, and that different brain parts work together to bring about the observable results. For example, different regions of the brain process letter groups which are not words, letter groups which have the form but which are not words, and letter groups which are words. Beyond this, different regions process different parts of speech such as nouns and verbs. Another example is involved with the perception of pain in which three distinct regions of the brain must function to enable one to perceive the pain, recognize its location, and its intensity.

Using EEG or brain wave tracings, E. Roy John, at the New York Medical College, claims to be able to identify specific regions of the brain involved in various rehabilitative and educational tasks such as oral reading, silent reading, paper and pencil arithmetic computations, mental computations, writing, etc. and to provide guidance for remediating different specific learning disabilities. He also claims that on the basis of his approximately 15-minute evoked analysis, he can estimate I.Q.s, as accurately as an intelligence test administered by a trained psychologist.

Very few studies using these kinds of techniques have been conducted with visually impaired children. This could be done from within the framework of a psychology of blindness which would not only benefit those with vision loss, but could assist in the broader aspects of psychology. For example, it is a well-established fact that some blind persons are capable of high levels of independent travel, while others get lost in a closet. It would seem instructive to compare brain processing in contrasting groups of blind travelers to identify whether different brain regions are functioning in these subjects, with possible means for stimulating lower functioning areas for greater potential. Good and poor Braille readers could be similarly studied with equally positive potential consequences.

Although there have been efforts made by some sociologists, as mentioned earlier, little actual research dealing with the social psychology of blindness has been conducted. Some studies cited in earlier chapters have noted differences in attitudes among educators and employers comparing the blind and other disability groups. The authors have not been able to find research which evaluates the impact, if any, a blind child exerts on a group of sighted children such as the presence of a visually impaired child in a regular classroom. Another potential social psychological area for research would relate to characteristics of organizations of the blind. What factors influence some blind persons to join with other blind persons to form some level of community, and others who prefer to find their community outside such a group? Which of these two groups has, on average, the better self-concept, self-esteem, and poorer attitudes toward blindness? Recently completed research by Kelly Poplawski has shown that visually impaired persons are significantly more likely to manifest symptoms of depression than the general public. Certain social factors such as marital status, employment and financial security mediate this tendency. It is one thing to note these statistical relationships and quite another to understand what social and psychological dynamics underlie the findings. Again, a psychology of blindness focus in research could offer help in understanding the processes involved.

It can be argued that all the research ideas suggested in this chapter could be conducted within the framework of nonpsychology-of-blindness circles. This is true. But will it be done? If it were to be done within the broader framework, implications and comparisons for other aspects of research could be reduced. There is certainly no philosophical imperative which would lead to specialized psychological foci. If the broader, more generic approach could be modified so systematic findings of importance for those working with the visually impaired could be developed, there is much which could be gained. However, the more nomothetic approach has tended to overlook contributions which could derive from focusing on specific subgroups.

A generic approach might prove useful for understanding the problems of the visually impaired if the underlying assumptions were not so restrictive as in most research. For example, if one were to observe a blind person in an unfamiliar environment, the observable behaviors would not be very helpful in understanding the situation. If one were to assume that it is possible to study feelings, intentions, and perseverance as these relate to vision loss, and if verbal reports provided by the subject were included as part of the data, information useful for more general problems of spatial orientation and a host of other issues might be found.

DISCUSSION

Efforts made to study the special and unique needs of the visually impaired need not be divisive. In fact, findings from studies of other groups such as the deaf and hard of hearing should be searched for ideas which have relevance for professional work assignments. Certainly research on any specialized interests can have meaning only as it is compared and contrasted with findings from the general fields of education and psychology. Studies based on a psychology of blindness would be able to make contributions for other disciplines in other fields in a reciprocal fashion.

The descriptions of "specialist" and "generalist" might guide us toward a more moderate book. "Specialists" are those who learn more and more about less and less until they know almost everything about practically nothing. "Generalists" are those who learn less and less about more and more until they know almost nothing about practically everything.

As with all endeavor there is probably some contribution to be made by both specialists and generalists. The authors hope this book will encourage all who read it to recognize the value of extensive study of the psychological impact of blindness or severe low vision on individuals of all ages. Greater understandings of how to serve those who are blind or who have low vision can be achieved through recognition of the necessity of inductive thinking processes as well as that individuals act on internal factors such as intention, motivation, etc. Hopefully, this book has discussed issue that incite professionals in work for the blind to provide better and more consistent services.

SUGGESTED READINGS

1. Hayes, S.P. (1941, 1971). *Contributions to a psychology of blindness.* New York: American Foundation for the Blind.
2. Kirtley, D.D. (1975). *The psychology of blindness.* Chicago: Nelson Hall.
3. Fraiberg, S. (1977). *Insights from the blind: Comparative studies of blind and sighted infants.* New York: Basic Books.
4. Lowenfeld, B. (1971). *Our blind children: Learning and growing with them.* Springfield, IL: Charles C Thomas.

LIST OF SUGGESTED READINGS

The following list of suggested readings provides a single place to look for citations given at the end of each chapter. In most cases specific pages are not specified in the hope that readers will look for more than a simple quote, but will give thoughtful consideration to the overall contribution each author has made to the field of work for the blind and visually impaired. Often the work of these and other pioneers in the field are regarded as "out of date" and their contribution is lost becaue of current "fads." It is hoped that reconsideration of earlier works will revive previous viewpoints and contribute toward study and research based on a psychology of blindness.

Barker, R.G. (1953). Adjustment to physical handicap and illness: A survey of the social psychology of physique and disability. *Social Science Research Council Bulletin, 55.*

Bateman, B.D. (1962). *Reading and psycholinguistic processes of partially sighted children.* Urbana-Champaign, IL: University of Illinois Press.

Bateman, B. (1965). Psychological evaluation of blind children. *New Outlook for the Blind, 59,* 193–196.

Bauman, M. K., & Yoder, N. M. (1966). *Adjustment to blindness reviewed.* Springfield, IL: Charles C Thomas.

Bishop, V.E. (2004). *Teaching visually impaired children* (3rd ed.). Springfield, IL: Charles C Thomas.

Board of Education of the Hendrick Hudson Central School Dis- trict, Westchester County et al. v. Rowley by her Parents Rowley et.us. U.S. Supreme Court No. 80–1002 June 28, 1982.

Bradley-Johnson, S. (1986). *Psycho-educational assessment of visually impaired and blind students preschool through high school.* Austin, TX: Pro-Ed.

Cholden, L.S. (1958). *A psychiatrist works with blindness.* New York: American Foundation for the Blind.

Cratty, B.J. (1967). The Perception of gradient and the veering tendency while walking without vision. *Research Bulletin,* American Foundation for the Blind, *14,* 31–51.

Cutsforth, T.D. (1951). *The blind in school and society.* New York: American Foundation for the Blind.

Ferrell, K.A. (1985). *Reach out and teach.* New York: American Foundation for the Blind.

Flinders, N. (1990). *Teach the children: An agency approach to education.* Provo, UT: Mormon Research Foundation.

Fraiberg, S., Siegel, B., & Gibson, R. (1966). The role of sound in the search behavior of a blind infant. *Psychoanalytic Study of the Child, 21,* 327–357.

Fraiberg, S. (1977). *Insights from the blind: Comparative studies of blind and sighted infants.* New York: Basic Books.

Gregory, R. L. (1997). *The eye and brain: The psychology of seeing.* (5th ed.). Princeton, NJ: Princeton University Press.

Hadley School for the Blind. (1986). *Knowing the system.* Winnetka, IL: Hadley School.

Hart, V. (1974). *Beginning with the handicapped.* Springfield, IL: Charles C Thomas.

Hayes, S.P. (1941, 1971). *Contributions to a psychology of blindness.* New York: American Foundation for the Blind.

Hebb, D.O., & Thompson, W.R. (1954). The social significance of animal studies. G. Lindsay & E. Arouson (Eds.), *The handbook of social psychology,* vol. 2 (2d ed.). Boston: Addison-Wesley, pp. 729-774.

Kirtley, D.D. (1975). *The psychology of blindness.* Chicago: Nelson Hall.

Koestler, Francis A. (1976). *The unseen minority: A social history of blindness in the United States.* New York: David McKay Company, Inc.

Lowenfeld, B. (1971). *Our Blind Children; Learning and Growing with Them.* Sp;ringfield, IL: Charles C Thomas.

Luterman, D.M., Melrose, J., Welsh, R.L. (1963). Auditory response in selected elderly men. *Journal of Gerontology, 18,* 267–280.

Miller, G. (1956). The magical number seven, plus or minus two: Some limits on our capacity for processing information. *Psychological Review, 63,* 81–97.

Penfield, W. *Speech and brain mechanisms.* Princeton, NY: Princeton University Press.

Piaget, J. (1952). *The origins of intelligence in children.* New York: International Universities Press.

Plutchik, R. (1980). *Emotions, a psychoevolutionary synthesis.* New York: Harper & Row.

Pribram, C. (1971). *Language of the brain: Experimental paradoxes in neural psychology.* New York: Prentice-Hall.

Russell, R.W. (1992). *To catch an angel: Adventures in a world I cannot see.* Vanguard Press.

Stephens, B., & Simpkins, K. (1974). The reasoning, moral judgment, and moral conduct of the congenitally blind: Final Project Report, H23-3197. Washington, DC: Office of Education, Bureau of Education for the Handicapped.

Stevens, G.D. (1962). *Taxonomy in special education for children with body disorder: The problem and a proposal.* Doctoral Dissertation. Columbia University, New York, NY.

Scholl, G.T. (1986). *Foundations of education for blind and visually handicapped children and youth: Theory and practice.* New York: American Foundation for the Blind.

Scholl, G. T., & Schnur, R. (1976). *Handbook for measurement and evaluation of the visually impaired.* New York: American Foundation for the Blind.

Thomas, G.E. (1992). *Mainstreaming, Are there any ill effects?* unpublished paper. Brigham Young University, Provo, UT.

Toffler, A. (1974). *Future shock—Learning for tomorrow: The roll of the future in education.* New York: Random House.

Toffler, A. (1980). *The third wave.* New York: Morrow.

Tuttle, D. (2004). *Self-esteem and adjusting with blindness* (3rd ed.). Springfield, IL: Charles C Thomas.

Warren, D. (1984). *Blindness and early childhood development.* New York: American Foundation for the Blind.

Welsh, R.L., & Blasch, B.B. (eds.). *Foundations of orientation and mobility.* New York: American Foundation for the Blind.

White, R. (1959). Motivation reconsidered: The concept of competence. *Psychological Review, 66*(5):297–333.

Wilber, L. (1937). *Vocations for the visually handicapped.* Oxford: American Foundation for the Blind.